*Emergencies*
in General Practice

# *Emergencies* in General Practice

**Dr A. J. Moulds,**
MB, ChB, FRCGP, DObst, RCOG

**Dr P. B. Martin,**
MBBS, FRCGP

**Col. T. A. I. Bouchier-Hayes,**
MB, ChB, FRCGP, DRCOG, RAMMC (Retd)



**Fourth Edition**

PETROC PRESS

*Petroc Press,* an imprint of LibraPharm Limited

**Distributors**
Plymbridge Distributors Limited, Plymbridge House, Estover Road, Plymouth PL6 7PZ, UK



First edition published 1983 by MTP Press Limited
Second edition 1987
Third edition 1993

Fourth edition published 1999 by
LibraPharm Limited, Suites 29–32, Venture West, New Greenham Park, NEWBURY, Berkshire, RG19 6HX, UK

Reprinted 2003

A catalogue record for this book is available from the British Library

ISBN 1 900603 86 1

Printed and bound in the United Kingdom by
Cromwell Press, Aintree Avenue, Trowbridge, Wilts BA14 0XB

# Contents

# Preface

This book has been written to provide general practitioners with an easy to read, easy to consult guide, to aid in the management of the large majority of practice emergencies.

Each presenting problem is approached logically with telephone assessment and advice followed by the assessment and management necessary when the patient is seen.

The emphasis is on practical primary care with discussion of differential diagnosis only taken as far as is needed for deciding the best immediate course of action. Words are kept to a minimum though tables are liberally used to summarise useful information. For each situation the final management advice is highlighted by being presented within a heavily lined box.

Our guiding principles for emergency care, which this book naturally reflects, are:

(1) When in any doubt—see the patient.
(2) Use the opportunity to educate by: explaining in simple language; not prescribing unless really necessary giving advice about managing everyday problems and about when it is important to call the doctor.

To use this book for ready reference by the telephone, in the car, or at the bedside:

(i) If the patient is a child, look at the contents list at the beginning of Chapter 4 and then turn to the relevant pages.
(ii) If the patient is an adult, first decide the system involved then look at the contents list at the beginning of the appropriate chapter before turning to the relevant pages.

*Acknowledgements*
We should like to record our grateful thanks to Mrs Nicola L. Moulds BSc for so expertly typing our manuscript. We should also like to thank the many doctors who have taken the time and the trouble to comment on the earlier editions of this book. In particular we should like to thank Dr Ben Essex and Dr Keith Hopcroft for their most helpful criticism.

# 1 Emergencies in Practice

In theory, every GP is responsible for his or her patients 24 hours a day, 7 days a week and every week of the year. However, on-call commitments vary greatly; from the single-handed rural GP with very little time off, to the urban practitioner who relies heavily on a local cooperative or deputising service and perhaps does only a few token night duties in the year. Whatever the actual time spent on call, every GP has to be prepared to deal with all manner of conditions outside the relative security and comfort of the surgery.

Emergencies provide only a small percentage of the GP's total workload. However, they generate a lot of emotional tension in patients and their relatives. They can also generate a lot of emotional tension in the doctor, who may feel insecure or cross at being disturbed, either in or out of 'normal' working hours, for what seems to be a trivial problem. Handling these situations with tact, skill and kindness pays great dividends. The doctor who is seen to be helpful will be trusted. If he or she then wishes to teach patients about self help or the appropriate use of emergency services, they will be more likely to listen.

Studies of 'out-of-hours' calls show, time and again, that the large majority of calls are either genuine medical emergencies or for conditions which have quite understandably produced anxiety in callers who, after all, are not medically qualified. Few calls are entirely unnecessary (4–15%), although the irritation that they can engender is disproportionate to their number. Most GPs find trying to deal with an urgent call whilst in the middle of a surgery very stressful.

In situations where the doctor cannot readily understand why the call has been made, exploring the caller's anxieties and fears is likely to be much more productive than a symptom-orientated cross-examination. For example, a child with a mild headache may be presented because of a family history of meningitis, or a baby with minor symptoms may be presented because of a sibling's cot death. Asking callers what it is that is really worrying them may well reveal hidden fears that can be allayed by telephone or by a, then acceptable, attendance at the surgery or primary care centre or visit. In many situations, it is the caller rather than the patient who needs reassurance or explanation. If this is not recognised, some problems will not be satisfactorily resolved.

GPs see an emergency early in its development, when symptoms and signs may be atypical. The doctor trained for hospital medicine often finds the transition to general practice traumatic because he or she is faced with problems that have not already been screened by another doctor. Management decisions have to be made without the supporting services or investigations that the hospital doctor is used to. It is vital to realise that while accurate diagnosis is satisfying it is not always possible, and it is perfectly legitimate to have a plan of action for a problem whose exact cause cannot be determined. In general, correct disposal is far more important than correct diagnosis. If doubt exists as to the correct disposal, the doctor must be prepared to see the patient again and reconsider or, at the least, to ensure that a responsible relative clearly understands under what circumstances the doctor should be contacted again.

Established practitioners may be at an advantage in knowing the patient and patient's family over many years. This may help in understanding reactions to illness and deciding appropriate action. However, it may also lead to prejudice or bias, which could result in an inappropriate and dangerous reaction.

## Who Does the Emergency Work

During normal working hours practices will cope with urgent calls. What is important is that surgery staff know how to handle the calls and know which doctor will deal with patients who need the advice of a doctor or who need to be seen. This means that staff must have written guidelines and a duty doctor rota so that they do not have to trawl through different partners to get a response.

For out of hours work there is an increasing tendency for GPs to farm out their obligations to commercial deputising services or to enrol in co-ops. A problem with co-ops is that you may have to do your fair share of shifts and these can be exhausting because you may be on call for large numbers of potential patients. That said, however, most GPs find that membership of a co-op transforms their life for the better.

Whatever system is used, the GP has to ensure that the doctor on call can deliver a quality service to the patients of the practice. It is important that efforts to educate patients are not undermined by deputising doctors and that problems are dealt with in a courteous and efficient manner. A dysfunctional emergency service is a quick way to alienate practice patients.

## When and Where to See the Patient

GPs have no legal obligation to see a patient or to visit purely on the demand of a patient or caller. Evidence of medical need allows the GP to decide whether the patient needs to be seen – we use the word seen as shorthand for urgent surgery or primary care centre consultation, or a home visit.

The doctor is also entitled to decide, on the basis of the information he or she has gathered, both when and where he or she will provide medical care. Under a GP's terms of service, the doctor's actions are judged by what his or her peers would compositely be expected to do or achieve; consensus rules.

When the surgery or primary care centre is open and staffed all the resources are available to deal with urgent problems. If callers can be assured that the patient will be seen reasonably quickly most will agree to a surgery consultation, if transport is available. This is a more rational and efficient way to provide care and is less stressful for the GP on call.

If the GP decides a child needs to be seen, but the parents refuse to bring the child out and insist on a visit, then the defence societies advise that the GP should visit. The child is the patient and should not be put in danger because of the unreasonable behaviour of the parents.

## Excerpts from the Terms of Service

***General***

3. Where a decision whether any, and if so what, action is to be taken under these terms of service requires the exercise of professional judgement, a doctor shall in reaching that decision not be expected to exercise a higher degree of skill, knowledge and care than GPs as a class may reasonably be expected to exercise.

***Service to Patients***

13. Subject to paragraph 3, a doctor shall render to his patients all necessary and appropriate personal medical services of the type usually provided by general medical practitioners. He shall do so at his practice premises or, if the condition of the patient so requires, elsewhere in his practice area or at the place the patient was residing when accepted by the doctor, or, if a patient was on the list of a practice declared vacant, when the doctor succeeded to that vacancy, or at some other place where the doctor has agreed to visit and treat him if the patient's condition so requires, and has informed the patient and the committee accordingly. The doctor shall not be required to visit and treat the patient at any other place. Such services include arrangements for referring patients as necessary to any other services provided for under the Health Service Acts and advice to enable them to take advantage of the local authority social services.

    This paragraph shall not impose an obligation on the doctor to provide contracep-tive services nor, except in an emergency, maternity medical services unless he has undertaken to provide such services.

A purely legalistic interpretation of these terms is not enough, as we have a moral obligation to provide care and patients with genuine anxieties are involved.

General practice provides continuing medical care for patients and their families and an abrasive, irritable approach while handling 'out-of-hours' or other urgent calls is a certain way to lose patients' confidence and respect. Patients will forgive almost anything, provided their doctor maintains a friendly attitude towards them. We cannot emphasise strongly enough that the guiding principles must always be:

---

(a) WHEN IN ANY DOUBT – SEE THE PATIENT
(b) SEE THE PATIENT FIRST – ARGUE OR EDUCATE LATER

---

In cases where telephone advice is the most appropriate initial action, it is worthwhile making clear to the caller that if the advice is not helpful or if symptoms change, another call will result in the patient being seen. The knowledge that the doctor will see the patient if simple measures do not help often gives callers confidence to manage the patient effectively without feeling that they have been forced to cope by an unwilling or unhelpful doctor. It also ensures that if the doctor has somehow misjudged the situation initially there will be a second chance to sort it out without the patient being taken direct to hospital or deteriorating at home while the relatives pluck up courage to call again.

Advice may be more safely given when the doctor knows that the patient can be told to come to an early appointment. Practices with appointment systems booked up for days ahead either have to leave specific appointments free for emergency cases or accept higher emergency visit rates as patients appreciate that they can only be seen reasonably quickly by demanding a visit.

In this book, we give a guide to when we think patients should be seen and when we think telephone advice is more appropriate. We have tried not to be overcautious but, of necessity, have erred on the side of seeing rather than telephone diagnosing and advising.

Paediatric emergencies are considered in a separate chapter (p. 15), whilst all adult emergencies are grouped in their appropriate system chapters. The emphasis is on practical primary care, and discussion of differential diagnosis is pursued only in so far as it is necessary for deciding the best immediate course of action.

The subject-matter layout is designed to allow presenting problems to be looked up quickly. A decision on the system involved can be followed by a glance at its chapter contents and the reading of the relevant pages.

On those occasions where a visit is necessary it may be worthwhile collecting a patient's notes from the surgery before visiting, particularly if the doctor does not know the patient and the case sounds as if it may be a little complicated. Good notes should be kept of the visit or consultation, regardless of whether the patient's records are available, and the usual records should be updated as soon as reasonably possible.

If there is no-one in when the doctor calls, it is more likely that the address has been taken down wrongly than that the patient has gone out. A note should be left stating the time of the call, and the original message taken should be carefully checked to see if any error has occurred.

## Admission of Patients to Hospital

This is most unlikely to pose problems. However, situations can arise where the GP requests hospital admission, but cannot get a bed. The responsibility for pursuing the matter rests squarely on the GP's shoulders and, having tried and failed, he or she cannot give up without exploring every available avenue.

Other hospitals in the area may have a bed, or the medical referee of an Emergency Bed Bureau may be able to help. If not, and it was a junior hospital doctor who refused admission, the consultant responsible should be contacted. The consultant who agrees that an admission is essential can be expected to help find a bed, if necessary in another hospital.

When the consultant agrees that admission is essential but cannot find a bed, then, according to the DoH, the GP should draw the attention of the RHA to the deficiencies in its services.

It must be rare to reach this stage, and the time involved is of little value to the patient who needs hospital care and the doctor's other patients who may also need attention. If the patient has to stay at home, an urgent domiciliary visit may well be indicated.

Alternatively in a real emergency the GP may be forced to advise the relatives to dial 999 and get the patient taken directly to hospital. There appropriate treatment can be instituted until a bed is found.

## Notes

# 2 Answering the Telephone

The era when the GP or his/her spouse had to field all the out of hours calls has now gone. Large rotas, coops and deputising services have trained staff who can take messages, give simple advice and make decisions about priorities. Nurses are often employed in this role and in some centres will also see patients and carry out triage to identify those needing a doctors opinion.

Even those GPs working in rural areas may be able to transfer calls to commercial answering services based many miles away. This can have a remarkably liberating effect on the GP and his/her family without diminishing the quality of the service to the patient.

During normal working hours surgery staff are the points of first contact and they must be trained to recognise serious problems and to handle distressed callers. Having trained their staff, some practices might consider employing them during evenings and weekends to take more of the stress out of emergency work.

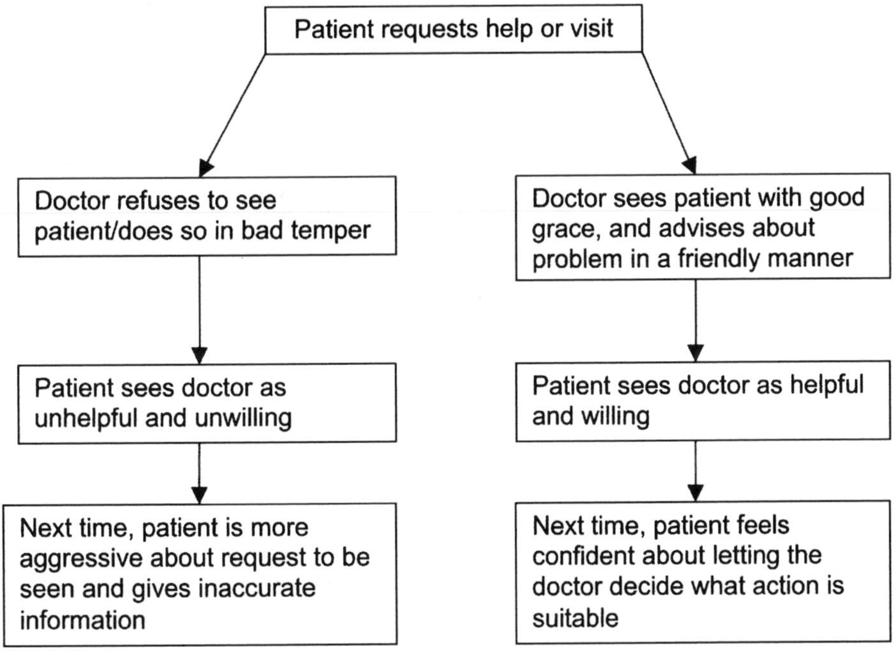

As nearly all requests for emergency or urgent care are made by telephone, this primary contact is very important because the way in which it is handled may have a considerable effect on the management both of the presenting problem and on future problems. A little care and consideration at this stage can pay great dividends later on.

Showing that you are willing to help will improve your relationship with patients and may actually help to reduce workload. If patients have found doctors to be unhelpful and unwilling to see them in the past, they may well be aggressive or feel the need to elaborate the story to ensure that they get action from the doctor. However, if they know that the doctor will definitely see them when it is necessary, they will be more willing to give accurate information and let the doctor decide what action is appropriate.

## Reasons for Telephoning

The decision to telephone for advice or for a patient to be seen or visited may be made by the patient, or by relatives or friends. Occasionally, other people (the milkman, the postman or the neighbours) may become aware of a problem and seek help from a doctor, with or without the patient's consent. The less willing a person is to accept responsibility, the more likely he or she is to call the doctor when faced with a difficulty.

If a family is tense or unstable, they will not be able to tolerate the extra anxiety generated by an illness. Similarly, people who are feeling guilty about not loving or looking after a relative are very likely to call a doctor in an effort to prove that they really do care.

Sometimes, the person who is presented as the patient is really not the patient at all. For instance, recurrent calls to see mildly ill children may be caused by depression in the mother.

Marital strife is quite a frequent cause of late calls. When father comes home from work or the pub and finds that one of the children is not well, he may call the doctor in an effort to make his wife look incompetent or negligent.

Always look for other reasons when a call seems to be inappropriate. Accept, however, that the vast majority of requests for advice or visits are made because of genuine anxiety.

## Accessibility

Worried patients find it difficult to cope with extra problems. Complicated telephone referral systems or telephone answering machines may be too much for them. They may give up or go to the local A & E department. Inaccessibility, whether intentional or not, is not a legitimate way of restricting your workload.

Where practical a single telephone number should be used for patients to contact the practice in an emergency. If taped messages are used they should be of good quality, easily understood and contain clear instructions.

### Information Needed

First, make sure that you get the name and address of the patient, as patients often assume that you know where they live. If the call is from a public kiosk, take a note of the number as the caller's money may run out prematurely.

Callers are looking for help and reassurance so it is important to signal the fact that you mean to be helpful early on. If you can say something like "of course I will see him if it is necessary but I need some information to find out what is needed", this will indicate to the caller that you are not putting up barriers. Further questioning is then likely to be seen as helpful rather than defensive.

Use simple language. Do not say 'Is his respiration distressed?'. 'Is he finding it difficult to breathe?' is better. Collect only the information that is necessary for you to decide:

1. Whether a visit is necessary
2. If it is necessary, how quickly and is any extra equipment or help needed?
3. If it is not necessary, is some other action more appropriate?

When in doubt, see the patient! Educate or discipline later.

## Appropriate Action

Advice may be the only action that is needed. Most patients accept this quite happily, although it is important to tell them to contact you again if the symptoms change or if they are worried for any other reason. Even if a patient only asks for advice, it is wise to ask yourself if they need to be seen or if a visit would be better. Any advice that you do give must be in simple language and should be easily understood and carried out.

If you decide that a visit is indicated, make sure you have got the address right. Ask for directions if you are not sure where the house is situated. This is particularly important where the house has a name but no number. Tell the caller roughly when you are likely to arrive.

In some emergencies, it may be more efficient to call an ambulance at once rather than visit and then call for help. Major trauma, burns, massive overdoses, myocardial infarctions and similar catastrophes are indications for a 999 call. Once you are involved it would be better for you to call the ambulance as the caller might be too confused to act appropriately. If you think you may be able to help in some way (by giving an analgesic, for example), go quickly, after calling the ambulance.

## Your Manner

Most patients are reasonable and considerate, but when worried and panicky they may appear abrupt and demanding. Bear this in mind and do not react too quickly. If necessary, take them to task after you have dealt with the problem. Keeping calm and friendly, even in the face of provocation, will enable you to get the information you need and to make your decisions more efficiently.

## Telephone Action Summary

1. Obtain the patient's name, address, telephone number, and doctor registered with.
2. Assess whether it is necessary to see the patient and if so where and when.

| *Necessary* | *Not necessary* |
|---|---|
| Assess the degree of urgency | 999 call better? |
| Is any extra equipment needed? | Advise in simple terms |
| Decide where to see the patient. | Ensure that you will be called again if the symptoms change or if the caller/ patient is worried |
| If home visit get directions, advise likely time of arrival, and at night, advise leave house lights on | |

# 3 The Doctor's Bag

The traditional black bag is an indispensable part of the GP's public image. The contents of a well-planned bag are essential for the provision of effective patient care.

Each doctor must decide what range of equipment and drugs he or she requires ready access to, to deal unaided with his or her practice's emergencies. Considerations such as the location and size of the practice area, the distance to the nearest hospital, the availability of local A & E services, likely ambulance response times and whether the practice provides a home obstetric service or routine care at road traffic accidents will all help determine what equipment is required and its disposition between the bag, the car boot and the surgery.

To avoid too many ifs and buts, and too intimidating a list of recommended drugs and equipment, we have confined ourselves to managing emergencies with a well stocked standard-sized bag. The only item of equipment we recommend which will not fit into the bag is a Volumatic or Nebuhaler with soft mask for use in the treatment of asthma. Those that prefer it may carry a nebuliser with them though we feel the large spacers are most convenient and many studies have shown them to be as effective as nebulisers. We do not include equipment for procedures like packing the nose and other activities which we feel are best attempted in the surgery or A & E rather than at home. Neither do we include lists of specialised equipment for obstetric care or accident management, as we are sure that the small minority or GPs involved in these activities know their own needs far better than we do.

For urban GPs, the only additional pieces of equipment that might be desirable are portable oxygen and IV infusion sets for use when ambulance response times are likely to be poor. For rural GPs without A & E back-up and with accident responsibility, much 'surgery' equipment will have to be carried in the car boot for the rare but vital times it may be needed. Of course, all GPs can pick up from the surgery equipment that they only very occasionally might want to use at home.

Also practices or coops need to agree a protocol about how they are to handle possible myocardial infarction. In urban areas, where ambulances equipped with paramedics and defibrillators are near at hand and hospital is only a few minutes away, the priorities are to get the patient to hospital quickly, ensure analgesia and administer oral aspirin. Where help is not so quickly available, GPs will have to consider whether they are going to administer thrombolytic drugs and whether the duty doctor should have a defibrillator and ECG to hand. This is a decision that would best be taken in conjunction with the local cardiologists.

Notwithstanding the needs of differing practices, it can be fairly stated that most emergency situations that arise are standard and, putting personal drug preferences aside, most GPs' bags should be interchangeable. The contents of our bag will allow for safe and effective management of virtually all the emergency situations GPs are likely to find themselves in.

## Basic Equipment

| | |
|---|---|
| Stethoscope | Assorted syringes and needles |
| Sphygmomanometer | Labstix |
| Ophthalmoscope and auriscope | Dextrostix |
| Thermometer | Soft Foley catheter (size 14–16) |
| Tendon hammer | Sterile dressings |
| Tongue depressors | Adhesive tape |
| Disposable gloves | Scissors |
| KY jelly | Brook type airways (adult/child) |
| Minims fluorescein 2% | Medicut (size 12–14) |
| Blood and urine test bottles | Mediswabs |
| | Volumatic and soft mask |
| | Mini peak flow meter |

## Stationery

| | |
|---|---|
| Continuation cards | Detailed map of practice area |
| Notepaper and envelopes | 20p piece for telephone |
| List of useful telephone numbers (see Appendix) | Forms for recommended emergency admission under the Mental Health Act (obtained from HM Stationery Office or local social work department) |
| MIMS or BNF | |
| Prescription pad | |
| National insurance and private certificates | |
| NHS claim forms for temporary residents | |

## Drugs

In the following tables and throughout the book, we have adopted a pragmatic approach to the naming of drugs. Where the generic name is in common usage and is easily recognised by the majority of GPs, we use it, but where we think the trade name is much more familiar, or where combination products are mentioned, we use the trade name. We accept that this is open to criticism, but we feel that it reflects the way GPs actually recognise drugs and use them in practice.

Please note that in both drug tables the dosages given are those of the standard preparation to be kept in the bag and are not necessarily the dose that will be prescribed.

For medico-legal reasons it is important you keep a record of the manufacturer and batch number of the drugs you use. If you have this product liability then lies with the manufacturer and not you.

## Locally Acting, Oral and Rectal Drugs

Paracetamol (tablet, 500 mg)
Dihydrocodeine tartrate (tablet, 30 mg)
Temgesic (buprenorphine; 0.2 mg; sublingual)

Penicillin V (sachets, 125 mg; tablet, 250 mg)
Erythromycin ethyl succinate (sachets, 125 mg and 250 mg)
Amoxil (amoxycillin sodium; capsule, 250 mg)
Trimethoprim (tablet, 100 mg)

Nitrolingual (GTN) spray x 1
Propranolol (tablet, 40 mg)
Frusemide (tablet, 40 mg)
Digoxin (tablet, 0.25 mg)
Soluble aspirin (tablet, 300 mg)

Salbutamol/inhaler x 2
Prednisolone (soluble tablet, 5 mg)
Phenergan (promethazine hydrochloride; tablet, 10 mg)

Haloperidol (Haldol; tablet, 5 mg)
Diazepam (tablet, 5 mg)
Stesolid rectal tube (diazepam; tube, 5 mg) x 4
Stemetil (prochlorperazine maleate; suppositories, 5 mg and 25 mg)

Hypostop x 1

Minims amethocaine 1%
Minims cyclopentolate 0.5%
Chloromycetin ointment 1% (chloramphenicol; 4 g tube)

## Parental Drugs

x 2 Cyclimorph 15 (morphine tartrate 15 mg, cyclizine tartrate 50 mg per 1 ml ampoule; SC or IM or IV)
x 2 Diclofenac (voltarol; 25 mg per ml; 3 ml ampoule; IM)
x 1 Amoxil (amoxycillin sodium; 500 mg powder in vial requiring 3 ml water for injection; IM or IV)
x 2 Benzylpenicillin (600 mg, corresponding to 1 mega unit powder in vial requiring 2 ml water for injection IM; or 4 ml for injection IV)
x 1 Chloramphenicol (IG requiring 2 ml water for injection IV or IM)

x 2 Atropine sulphate (0.6 mg in 1 ml ampoule)
x 1 Lignocaine 1% (20 ml vial)
x 2 Frusemide (50 mg in 5 ml ampoule)
x 3 Hydrocortisone sodium succinate (100 mg powder in vial requiring 1–2 ml water for injection; IV)

*Continued*

x 3 Haloperidol (Haldol; 10 mg in 2 ml ampoule;IM)
x 2 Diazemuls (Diazepam; 10 mg in 2 ml ampoule; IM, IV)
x 2 Stemetil (prochlorperazine maleate; 12.5 mg in 2 ml ampoule; IM)
x 1 Maxolon (metoclopramide hydrochloride; 10 mg in 2 ml ampoule; IM)

x 2 Adrenaline (Epinephrine; 1 in 1000 strength 0.5 ml ampoule; IM)
x 1 Piriton (chlorpheniramine maleate; 10 mg in 1 ml ampoule; SC or IM or slow IV)

x 1 Glucagon (1 unit in 1 ml vial to be dissolved in accompanying solvent; IM or SC or IV)

x 1 Syntometrine (0.5 mg ergometrine and 5 units synthetic oxytocin in 1 ml ampoule; IM)

x 1 Deltastab (prednisolone acetate; 25 mg per ml in 5 ml vial; intra articular or local injection)

x 5 Water for injection (2 ml ampoule)

NB: GPs in areas where IV drug abuse is a problem may wish to carry x 3 Naloxone (Narcan; 0.4 mg in 1 ml ampoule; SC or IM or IV)

## Prescribing Notes

- Except for the paediatric section, which has its own prescribing notes (see p. 17), all drug doses given throughout this book are standard adult does.
- Recommended doses may need to be varied for individual patients, particularly the elderly and those with hepatic or renal disease.
- All our prescribing advice is based on the assumption that the doctor will exclude drug allergy and other possible contraindications before administering a drug.
- We have theoretical and practical reasons for recommending the drugs we do, although the choice between drugs of similar pharmacological properties and equal effectiveness is a personal one.
- It is vital that the doctor should be familiar with the range of drugs he or she uses and any possible interactions between them.
- Very few callers do not have ready access to simple analgesics, cough medicines, antacids which can be taken in response to telephone or direct advice.
- Do not prescribe unless there are clear indications.
- Do not prescribe simple remedies that patients could reasonably be expected to buy for themselves. Prescribing for minor illnesses justifies the caller's belief that the doctor's attendance was necessary; non-prescribing helps to educate patients as to which illness can be self-managed in the future.
- Re-stock your bag after each spell on call, and fully revise and update its contents every 6 months, paying particular attention to drug expiry dates.

# 4 Paediatric Emergencies

*The presentation, diagnosis and management of acute illness in babies and children poses problems so different from those posed by adults that we felt the most logical and helpful way of discussing them was in a separate chapter of the book.*

*There is some cross-referral with the chapters dealing with the adult system, although our aim has been to make this chapter as self-contained as possible. It should provide advice that will help in the resolution of the large majority of paediatric emergencies.*

## Chapter Contents

For vomiting and diarrhoea, see 'The vomiting child', p. 35

See also Head injury, p. 112
See also Red eye, p. 86
See also Epistaxis, p. 80
See also Foreign body in the ear, p. 79
See also Foreign body in the nose, p. 82

## 4.1 Introduction

A considerable proportion of out-of-hours calls are made for acute illnesses in children. Many of the conditions are fairly trivial from a purely medical point of view, but parents, particularly those of fairly limited experience, may become very anxious about their children's symptoms. In these days of small families, people may grow up and start having their own children without ever having had the experience of looking after younger brothers and sisters. When they are suddenly faced with an ill child, they are understandably anxious and may have no older relative or friend near by, from whom they can get advice or reassurance. The result is usually a call to the doctor.

Good parents should be anxious about their children, and it is important for the doctor to be understanding and tolerant. If they see you as a kind person who wants to be helpful, they are less likely to be demanding and are more likely to take your advice if you think that the child does not need to be seen.

Remember that parents know the normal behaviour of their children. If they are sure that their child is ill, they are likely to be right, even if you cannot find anything wrong the first time you examine the child. Listen carefully to what the parents have to say and take them seriously. Do not say 'There is nothing wrong'. The parents are sure to be very resentful if the child eventually turns out to be ill. It is much more tactful to say that you cannot find evidence of any serious illness and that you are willing to see the child again, if necessary.

Some calls are made because the family is undergoing some psychosocial stress and the added anxiety of an intercurrent illness in a child just cannot be tolerated. In these circumstances, the call may be made in an aggressive or a demanding manner. The doctor must try to keep cool and deal with the clinical situation; there is a danger that this could be mishandled if anger is allowed to cloud clinical judgement. When the illness has been dealt with, the doctor can then attend to the problem of the aggression. The parents are usually very compliant once they see that the doctor is not taking risks with the health of their child. Firm advice that their child will get the attention that it needs and that, therefore, aggression is neither necessary nor acceptable, should improve future relationships. You should also indicate that you are sympathetic and willing to help with any psychosocial problem, if it is in your power to do so. This mixture of firmness and helpfulness will usually solve most of the difficulties that arise from these aberrant situations.

## 4.2 Paediatric Prescribing

Paediatric dosage schedules tend to be based on adult dosages, appropriately adjusted in terms of either body weight or surface area. In practice, it is easier to use the basis of body weight, although this may be incorrect if the child is obese. Details of the drugs which we use for the emergency care of children are given at the end of this section. When drugs are mentioned in the text, we may give no dosage details. If you have any doubts about the correct dose for the child's age, refer to the information at the end of this section.

Throughout the text, we take no account of possible contraindications or allergies that may exist; to do so would be boringly repetitious. Nevertheless, we must emphasise that you, the prescribing doctor, should always enquire about known drug allergies and always be aware of factors, such as renal or liver impairment, which might affect the drug or the dose that you should use.

### 4.2.1 Administration of drugs

The oral route is that normally used for most drugs, remembering that, for younger children, liquids are likely to be more easily administered than tablets. If a 5 ml syringe is not used then a standard level teaspoon is the correct 5 ml dosage measurement: household teaspoons are inaccurate in view of the wide variation in their capacity. Medicines should not be added to an infant's bottle, as then the whole dose may not be taken or there may even be an interaction with the milk.

Parents may have difficulty in getting children to take medicine. If a child clenches his teeth, drugs in liquid form may be given by placing the point of a small spoon or syringe down the side of the child's mouth (between teeth and cheek) to well behind the back teeth. A child's nose should not be held to try to force him to take medicine. He will certainly be even more resistant to taking further medicine and may even aspirate the drug.

If the child persistently refuses drugs or is vomiting, there is little point giving oral medication and the need for parenteral administration is indicated. Similarly, in ill children, parenteral administration may be appropriate initially as a means of achieving rapid therapeutic levels. IM injection should be given into the lateral aspect of the thigh or the deltoid area. IV injection should be given into the antecubital or other superficial veins. Venepuncture may be impossible in an uncooperative child or in a small baby, and a second-best route may have to be used. IV diazepam, for example, is the treatment of choice for a fitting child, but the difficulties of administering it may make the rectal route more practicable.

In general, the administration of drugs per rectum tends to be unreliable. Suppositories should be inserted into an empty rectum or they may be swiftly expelled in a faecal cocoon.

Administration of drops into the eyes, nose or ears of an obstreperous child may be best achieved by wrapping him in a blanket which restrains arm and leg movements.

Prescriptions left with parents should be accompanied with firm advice as to what exactly is required. The timing of doses is particularly important and should be spelt out.

## 4.3 Recommended Emergency Drugs

### 4.3.1 Paracetamol

- Analgesic and antipyretic effects as good as aspirin.
- No anti-inflammatory action.
- Can be given to children of any age, unlike aspirin.

- No absolute contraindications, but use with caution if there is liver or renal dysfunction.
- Side effects and adverse reactions rare.

Available as syrup (120 mg in 5 ml) and tablet (500 mg).

| *Age* | *Dose* |
|---|---|
| Less than 1 year | Syrup (2.5–5 ml) QID |
| 1–5 years | Syrup (5–10 ml) QID |
| 6–12 years | Syrup (10–20 ml) or half to one tablet (250–500 mg) QID |

### 4.3.2 Benzylpenicillin (Crystapen)

- In any patient with suspicion of bacterial meningitis an initial dose of parenteral penicillin given before admission to hospital improves the outcome.
- Dose is ideally given IV but if this is not possible then give IM.

| *Age* | *Dose* |
|---|---|
| Under 1 year | 300 mg |
| 1–9 years | 600 mg |
| 10 years + | 1200 mg |

- As a guide 1.2 g needs to be dissolved in 8 ml water if being given IV or 4 ml water if IM.
- If allergic to penicillin use chloramphenicol sodium succinate (1 g vial). The dose for adults is 1 g and children 12.5 mg/kg. Give IV or, if not possible, IM.

### 4.3.3 Penicillin V

- Antibiotic of choice when one is indicated for tonsillitis or otitis media in a child over 5 years.
- If child allergic to penicillin, use erythromycin.
- Best given before meals.
- May cause diarrhoea.

Available as syrup (125 mg in 5 ml) and tablet (125 mg and 250 mg).

| *Age* | *Dose* |
|---|---|
| Less than 1 year | 62.5 mg QID |
| 1–5 years | 125 mg QID |
| 5–10 years | 250 mg QID |

### 4.3.4 Erythroped (Erythromycin Ethyl Succinate)

- Non-toxic alternative when penicillin indicated, but hypersensitivity exists.
- Do not use in conjunction with other anti-infective agents.
- Few side effects, although may cause abdominal discomfort, nausea and vomiting.

- Allergic reactions rare.

Available as PI suspension (125 mg in 5 ml) and ordinary suspension (250 mg in 5 ml).

| *Age* | *Dose* |
|---|---|
| Less than 2 years | 125 mg QID |
| 2–8 years | 250 mg QID |
| 8 years and over | 500 mg QID |

### 4.3.5 Amoxil (amoxycillin)

- Broad-spectrum antibiotic for otitis media (in child under 5 years), chest and urinary tract infections.
- If child allergic to penicillin, use erythromycin for otitis media and chest infection, and trimethoprim for urinary tract infections.
- No absolute contraindications other than penicillin allergy.
- May cause diarrhoea or allergic rashes.

Available as syrup (125 mg in 5 ml), capsule (250 mg) and injection (250 mg).

| *Age* | *Dose* |
|---|---|
| Under 10 years | 125 mg TID (if severe infection, double dose) |
| Over 10 years | 250 mg TID (if severe infection, double dose) |

If oral route impractical, or urgent treatment for severe infection is necessary, give IM.

| | |
|---|---|
| Under 10 years | 250 mg dissolved in 1.5 ml water |
| Over 10 years | 500 mg dissolved in 3 ml water |

- If giving to a child who cannot swallow capsules, break capsule, mix contents with 2 teaspoonfuls of Ribena and give child one or two teaspoonfuls of the mixture.

### 4.3.6 Salbutamol (Ventolin)

- Selective beta 2 adrenergic stimulant for relief of bronchospasm.
- Few side effects, but may cause tremor and palpitations.
- Volumatic can be effectively used by younger children. It has been shown to be as effective as a nebuliser. With small children use with mask. Tilt upwards to make valve open more easily while child breathes in contents of chamber.

### 4.3.7 Diazepam (Diazemuls; Stesolid rectal tube)

- Use IV or rectally for status epilepticus.
- No contraindications, but IV should be given into a large vein of the antecubital fossa with the patient kept supine.

- Injection should be given slowly (0.5 ml of solution per half minute) until eyelids droop or fit stops.
- Rare possibility of apnoea or hypotension is much decreased if given in this manner.
- IV injection may produce thrombophlebitis but this is lessened by use of Diazemuls.
- In emergency, IV is probably only feasible in older children.
- If baby or young child is fitting, rectal route is likely to be best.
- IV solution given rectally in syringe without needle acts about 5 minutes later than same dose given intravenously.

Available as vial (10 mg in 2 ml) or rectal tube (5 mg)

| *Route* | *Dose* |
|---|---|
| Rectally | 1–3 years of age—one 5 mg tube inserted halfway to mark on nozzle<br>4 years or more—two 5 mg tubes<br>In both cases if no effect is seen after 5 minutes the same dose may be given again. |
| IV | 0.15–0.25 mg per kg body weight |

## 4.4 Child Abuse

- Always be on the lookout for evidence of physical or mental child abuse.

### Situations of Potential Child Abuse

- You are in a particularly good position to identify situations which may lead to child abuse.
- Remember the association of child abuse with
  - low birth weight babies
  - babies who have been separated from their mother soon after birth
  - young parents with social or personal difficulties
  - children repeatedly presented with crying, vomiting or feeding difficulties.
- Parents at the end of their tether may make unnecessary urgent calls and display anxiety, aggression or both.
- When you detect a lot of emotion, keep calm and ask the parents, in a sympathetic way, if they are getting so upset that they feel like hitting or shaking the child. They are often relieved to be able to talk about their feelings and will do so if they feel that you are on their side.

**Action when seen**

- **Assessment**
  - Be prepared to make a diagnosis of established child abuse in children who
    - are habitually dirty and unkempt

- are apathetic and behind in their development
- are repeatedly injured
- have injuries inconsistent with the story
- are presented some time after an alleged incident
- have multiple bruising, finger grasp marks or unusual lesions like cigarette burns
- have bruising on the face (this is seen in over 80% of abused children).

**● Management**

| *Assessment* | *Management* |
|---|---|
| Potential abuse | Offer maximum support from yourself, the health visitor and social services<br>If the situation is very tense, **admission** is fully justified to allow the crisis to cool off |
| Established abuse | **Admit,** ensuring that hospital staff know the real reason for admission<br>Initiate local protocol. |

## 4.5 Cot Death

- Will occur once every 4 years for the average GP.
- Generally occurs in babies 1–6 months old, from poor social background, during winter.
- In one third of cases the baby has serious abnormalities, in one third a significant illness and in one third the baby is well or suffering from only mild symptoms before death.
- By definition, cot death is unexpected and naturally causes tremendous anxiety, panic and guilt feelings in the parents.

**Visit**

**Action on arrival**

**● Management**

- Make sure that this is not an abused or murdered child.
- Inform the parents that a postmortem will be necessary.
- Warn that police will visit and explain why.
- Support the parents and give special help and understanding to all those involved to help relieve them of their inevitable guilt feelings.

**Before leaving**

- Arrange to see parents the next day in order to arrange ongoing care for them.
- Tell parents about the Foundation for Study of Infant Deaths who provide a 24 hour support line. Tel: 0171 253 1721.

## 4.6 The Crying Child

A fairly frequent reason for an emergency call, the crying child is a potent cause of anxiety and even anger in its parents. In young children, crying is the normal response to physical or emotional distress. The cause of this distress may not be apparent to the parents and even you may find difficulty in arriving at a definite diagnosis. Remember anxiety in the mother may make the baby anxious and irritable.

## 4.6.1 Crying of Acute Onset

- Severe crying or screaming in a normally happy infant is significant.
- May be difficult to obtain a clear history, because the parents are preoccupied with the screaming; the child must be seen.

**See**

**Telephone advice**

- *Try to keep calm. Give the baby a cuddle and I will see you shortly.*

**Action when seen**

- **Assessment**
  - Crying may be caused by any painful condition.
  - Take a careful history, including asking:
    - Has there been any preceding accident or illness?
    - Is the crying episodic?
    - Is the child worse when touched or moved?
    - Does the child draw up his or her legs?
    - Is the distress associated with attempts to defaecate or micturate?
  - Undress the child completely and perform a full examination, feeling all over for tenderness or pain on movement.
  - Pay particular attention to the examination of the ears, abdomen and genitalia.
  - If the crying has no very obvious cause, consider the possibility of meningitis.

| *Commoner causes* | *Features* |
|---|---|
| Otitis media | Commonest cause<br>URTI and child febrile with red bulging ear-drums.<br>(Do NOT diagnose if ear-drums are only slightly inflamed) |
| Abdominal pain or colic | Drawing up the legs<br>Child pale during an attack<br>Bowel symptoms or abnormal abdominal examination |
| Osteomyelitis | Child febrile<br>Tender over a bone<br>NB: May not be much tenderness or swelling early on |
| Fracture | May be history of trauma |

*Continued*

| *Commoner causes* | *Features* |
|---|---|
| | Child keeps limb still<br>Tender over the bone<br>NB: Consider the possibility of child abuse |
| Strangulated hernia | Tender swelling in inguinal or umbilical area |
| Torsion of testicle | Tender swollen scrotum |
| Inflamed foreskin | Child screams upon attempting to micturate |
| Inflamed perianal area | Recent diarrhoea or monilial nappy rash<br>Pain worse when attempting to defaecate |

- **Management**
  - Diagnose and treat the underlying condition.
  - If you find no cause and the crying persists, **admit** for observation.

## 4.6.2 The Always Crying Child

- Not really a medical emergency, but parents may have reached the end of their tether, especially if faced with the prospect of another sleepless night.
- Explosive situation with much anger generated: 'There must be something wrong with him'.
- Could lead to baby-battering.
- Characteristically, baby is otherwise well, feeding properly and gaining weight.
- Parents may telephone for advice only, but it may be better to see the child, give reassurance and dissipate the anxiety and anger which may put the child at risk.

**See**

**Action when seen**

- **Assessment**
  - Carefully examine the baby to
    - exclude the possibility of significant illness
    - assess the baby's standard of care
    - reassure the parents.
  - Talk to the parents to decide
    - how competent they are
    - what social, marital or other problems they have
    - whether they feel that they could hit or shake the baby in their frustration.
  - If possible watch the parents giving a feed; you can learn a lot from this.

- **Management**

| *Assessment* | *Management* |
|---|---|
| Baby not at risk | Firmly reassure that the baby is normal<br>Firmly reassure that they are not bad parents<br>If you are good at handling babies, give it a cuddle or even a feed<br>Offer continued support from yourself or a health visitor |
| Baby at risk and/or parents not coping | **Admit** |

## 4.7 The Feverish Child

- Although other symptoms often indicate the cause, it is the fever that usually worries the parents.
- Consider the likely cause of the fever and the likely risk of a febrile convulsion.
- Ask about other symptoms and try to determine how ill the child is. Is the child in bed, irritable or not eating properly?

**See if**

- this is a young child, especially under 2 years
- there is a history of febrile convulsions
- there is no obvious cause for the fever
- there is a possible serious cause for the fever
- child has a very high temperature
- fever has been present for more than 24 hours
- child is irritable or unusually drowsy
- parents are anxious and clearly need reassurance.

**Telephone advice**

- When no need to see
  *Fever is the body's response to infection, and in itself it is not dangerous. Keep the child cool and lightly clothed. Encourage a high fluid intake. Use paracetamol only if the fever is interfering with sleep. Call me again if the child gets worse or develops new symptoms.*

- Before seeing the child
  *If the child is at risk of a febrile fit, sponge it down with tepid water and give paracetamol syrup. Do not put the child in the bath or use cold water. I will see you shortly.*

**Action when seen**
**Assessment**

- Take careful history and perform full examination to try to establish cause.
- NB: Teething is not a cause.
- If no obvious ENT or respiratory infection, consider the possibility of UTI or meningitis.

- Do not forget malaria if the child has recently been abroad.
- Risk of febrile fit if
  - fever is very high
  - child is twitchy or very irritable
  - past or family history of fits.

**Management**

| *Assessment* | *Management* |
|---|---|
| Mild fever<br>High fever with no distress | In all cases, treat the underlying condition appropriately<br>Do NOT use antibiotics unless they are obviously indicated<br>Dress child in cool clothing and maintain a high fluid intake |
| High fever with distress (i.e. irritability, loss of sleep, delirium) | Paracetamol every 4 hours<br>Sponge down with lukewarm water<br>Use a fan, if available<br>Maintain a high fluid intake |
| High risk of febrile fit | Advice as above<br>Stesolid 5 mg rectal tube:<br>1–3 years old one tube inserted halfway to mark on nozzle;<br>4 years or more—2 tubes. |
| Pyrexia of unknown origin | **Admit if**<br>● this is a small baby<br>● child obviously toxic<br>● fever has persisted for some days<br>**Home care if**<br>● older child<br>● fever has been of short duration<br>● child is otherwise well<br>Take MSU for culture<br>See again within 24 hours, sooner if the child worsens or new symptoms develop |

# 4.8 Respiratory Tract Infections in Children

## 4.8.1 General Telephone Assessment and Advice

- Respiratory tract infections are the commonest cause of out-of-hours calls.
- Reason for call is usually parental anxiety about the fever or pain associated with the infection.
- Less commonly, coughing or respiratory distress may be the presenting feature.
- Try to obtain enough information to decide whether or not a visit is indicated.

- If you are a high prescriber of antibiotics and cough linctuses, parents will phone you because you have conditioned them to expect treatment and they need a doctor to get the drugs.

| *Indications for* **telephone advice** | *Indications to* **see** |
|---|---|
| Little or no fever | High fever |
| Active child | Lethargic or weak child |
| No pain | Pain |
| Taking fluids and food | Not eating or drinking |
| Moderate cough | Severe cough which keeps child awake |
| No respiratory distress | Any signs of respiratory distress or history of underlying lung problem |
| Older child | Infants or young children |
| Good social conditions | Poor social conditions |
| Stable parents | Anxious or unstable parents |

**General telephone advice**

- When no need to see
  Explain that this is a virus infection, so antibiotics are not indicated.
  *No specific treatment is needed, but paracetamol suspension may be given 4 hourly if necessary for pain or fever. Solids are not as important as maintaining a high fluid intake. Tepid sponging can make the hot, cross child feel better. Make appointment for the next surgery if the child needs to be seen, e.g. for earache or sore throat. Call again if the child worsens or if any new symptoms develop.*
- Before seeing the child
  Advise as above, depending on how long you feel it will be before you need to see the child.

**Action when seen**

**● Assessment**

- Take routine history and perform examination to make an exact diagnosis and to assess the general condition of the child.
- Exclude serious diseases like meningitis or pneumonia.
- Decide whether there is any indication for the use of antibiotics.

## 4.8.2 Simple Febrile Cough and Cold

- Viral infection with no evidence of otitis media or chest involvement.

**● Management**

- Give simple advice on the use of household remedies.
- Do NOT give antibiotics.
- Avoid giving a prescription; this is an effective way of teaching parents that URTIs do not require medical intervention.

## 4.8.3 Acute Febrile Sore Throat

- At least 60% are viral: there is little way clinically to distinguish those which are streptococcal, although strawberry tongue, circumoral pallor or a scarlet fever rash would be suggestive.

**● Management**

| *Assessment* | *Management* |
|---|---|
| Child not ill | Maintain high fluid intake<br>Paracetamol every 4 hours |
| Child has high fever or is toxic | As above, plus penicillin V stat. and 5-day course |

## 4.8.4 Otitis Media

- May complicate any respiratory infection in children.
- Child under 2 years presents with persistent crying or screaming.
- Where clearly earache and child not toxic most can be dealt with on the telephone.

**See if**

- high fever
- child toxic or vomiting
- pain for more than 24 hours
- recurrent problem
- parents very anxious

**Telephone advice**

- When no need to see

  Give paracetamol 4 hourly if necessary. Antibiotics will not shorten the attack and are not indicated at this stage. If earache persists or a discharge develops then make appointment with your own doctor or call back.

**Action when seen**

**● Assessment**

- Examine ear-drums.
- Check for meningism and mastoid tenderness.

**● Management**

| *Assessment* | *Management* |
|---|---|
| Little or no fever<br>Mildly congested ear-drum<br>Ear-drum not pulsatile or perforated<br>No discharge<br>Pain less than 24 hours | Advise high fluid intake<br>Paracetamol elixir every 4 hours |
| Marked fever<br>Very red ear-drum<br>Ear-drum pulsatile or perforated<br>Discharge<br>Pain more than 24 hours | As above, plus Amoxil stat. and 3-day course |

**Before leaving**

- advise parents that if after 6 weeks they are at all suspicious that the child is deaf, they must bring him or her to the surgery for reassessment ± audiogram.

## 4.8.5 Acute Bronchitis

- May complicate any respiratory infection in children.
- Usually characterised by fever, cough and scattered coarse rhonchi.
- If the child is severely toxic or has any respiratory distress then the diagnosis is likely to be bronchopneumonia not bronchitis.

- **Management**

| *Assessment* | *Management* |
|---|---|
| Mild fever<br>White sputum<br>Child over 1 year<br>Good social conditions | High fluid intake<br>Simple cough linctuses, if you wish<br>Call again if the patient worsens or if new symptoms develop |
| High fever<br>Patient toxic<br>Coloured sputum<br>Child under 1 year<br>Poor social conditions | If admission not necessary as above, plus Amoxil stat. and 5-day course<br>See again in 24–48 hours |

**Before leaving**

- remember that all children with signs in their chests should be followed up to ensure that the chest clears.

## 4.8.6 Acute Bronchiolitis

- Acute respiratory syncytial virus infection in children usually less than 1 year old.
- Characterised by rapid-onset, fever, cough and wheeze. Infant toxic with respiratory distress, many rhonchi and creps.

- **Management**

- ADMIT (most are hypoxic).

## 4.8.7 Pneumonia

- Pneumonia of minor degree is not uncommon in children with respiratory tract infections.
- Often no physical signs in the early stages, so be prepared to re-examine the chest of a child with persistent cough.
- May be little systematic distress and few patches of creps., or serious illness with high fever and respiratory distress.
- *Remember* pain on respiration may be a cause of crying and basal pneumonia is a cause of abdominal pain.

● **Management**

| *Assessment* | *Management* |
|---|---|
| Older child<br>No respiratory distress<br>Not toxic | Give extra fluids |
| Minimal consolidation<br>Good social conditions | Amoxil stat. and 5-day course<br>See again within 24 hours<br>Consider postural drainage (instruct parents in this) |
| Infant or young child<br>Respiratory distress<br>Ill-looking or toxic child<br>Extensive consolidation<br>Poor social conditions | **Admit** |

**Before leaving**

- ensure that the parents will call if there is any deterioration – particularly if any breathing difficulty develops.
- advise the parents that a chest X-ray may be necessary later.

## 4.8.8 Croup and Stridor

- Croup usually describes the symptoms of acute laryngotracheobronchitis (i.e. explosive barking cough, hoarse voice, stridor).
- Stridor may also be caused by acute epiglottitis or inhalation of a foreign body.

| *Cause of stridor* | *Features* |
|---|---|
| Viral acute laryngotracheobronchitis | Child has usually had a cold for a few days<br>Child is usually fairly well, and can eat and drink<br>May be mildly febrile<br>Hoarse voice and barking cough are prominent symptoms<br>High-pitched stridor |
| Acute epiglottis | Explosive onset or history of sore throat rather than a cold<br>Cough not prominent<br>Child sits still and leans forward<br>Child febrile and toxic<br>Child drools saliva and finds swallowing painful<br>Soft, low-pitched stridor<br>Tachycardia: over 160 |

*Continued*

| *Cause of stridor* | *Features* |
|---|---|
| Inhalation of foreign body | No signs of infection<br>Until ruled out, regard unexpected spasm of coughing or stridor as being caused by an inhaled foreign body, even if the patient appears to be better when seen |

- Severity of the stridor is clinically important.

| *Very mild* | *Moderate* | *Severe* |
|---|---|---|
| Stridor only after a bout of coughing or crying | Some stridor present at rest | Constant stridor, which may even be expiratory |
| Child active | Child very anxious | Child lies quiet<br>May be drowsy |
| Good colour at all times | May become slightly blue during coughing | Grey or pale skin<br>Blue lips |
| Little or no use of accessory muscles | Use of accessory muscle during and after bouts of coughing | Marked use of accessory muscles |
| | Some intercostal recession | Severe intercostal recession |

- Child with croup is best assessed by observation rather than examination.
- Do NOT examine throat if you have the slightest suspicion of acute epiglottitis, as this may precipitate respiratory and cardiac arrest.
- Listen to the chest, although this is usually clear.

**Action when seen**

| *Assessment* | *Management* |
|---|---|
| ANY suspicion of epiglottitis | Do NOT examine throat<br>**Admit**—Go to hospital with the child |
| Croup with moderate stridor | **Admit** |
| ANY suspicion of an inhaled foreign body | **Refer** to A & E (see p. 164) |
| Croup with little stridor | Advise re inhalation of steam<br>Instruct parents to stay up with child<br>Ask to be recalled if the child worsens |

## 4.9 The Wheezy or Asthmatic Child

- Wheezing may be associated with any lower respiratory tract infection.
- Recurrent wheezy 'bronchitis' should be regarded as asthma, so that child is treated appropriately with bronchodilators, rather than inappropriately with antibiotics.

**See**
- if parents are worried about the child's breathing
- even if the child is a known asthmatic with medication at home.

**Telephone advice**
- Before seeing the child
  *If it has not been used already, give 2 puffs of the inhaler. I shall see you shortly.*

**Action when seen**

- **Assessment**
  - Degree of audible wheeze is not a good guide to the severity of the bronchospasm.

| *Mild bronchospasm* | *Severe bronchospasm* |
|---|---|
| Child up and about | Child lies or sits very still |
| Child may be cross | Child anxious rather than cross |
| Good colour | Pale skin, blue lips |
| Little or no use of accessory muscles | Maximum use of accessory muscles |
| Good air entry | Poor air entry (beware the silent chest) |

### 4.9.1 Up to 18 Months

- Wheezing likely to be bronchitis or bronchiolitis.
- May be a 'fat, happy' wheezer who is not ill.
- Neither are very responsive to bronchodilators until about 20 months.

- **Management**
  - Amoxil stat. and 5-day course (if chest infection present).
  - Try Salbutamol inhaler 2–4 puffs by Volumatic and mask.
  - If bronchiolitis or baby appears ill or distressed or ANY respiratory difficulty present. **Admit**

### 4.9.2 Eighteen Months and Older

- **Management**
  - Salbutamol inhaler 4 puffs by Volumatic. Use mask if child not cooperative. Repeat in 5–10 minutes if necessary.
  - If inhaler effective:
    Leave inhaler and advise parents to give 2 puffs 3 hourly, whether child wheezy or not, until child is seen again.
    Antibiotics only if there is good evidence of bacterial infection.

Consider whether short course oral prednisolone is needed or not (see below)

- If inhaler not effective give oral prednisolone start dose (see below) and **admit.**

**Before leaving**

- consider whether it is necessary to see again in a few hours
- advise parents to call if there is any relapse
- arrange for review, including long-term management.

### 4.9.3 The Recurrent Wheezer

- If bouts of persistent wheezing occur in spite of adequate bronchodilator therapy, use short course of steroids in addition to usual therapy. If necessary, leave enough tablets from bag for first doses. Give a 5 day course at dose shown below. There is no need to taper off short courses.

| *Age* | *Dose of prednisolone daily* |
|---|---|
| 1 | 15 mg |
| 3 | 20 mg |
| 5 | 25 mg |
| 7 | 30 mg |
| 10+ | 40 mg |

- Start inhaled prophylatic therapy e.g. Beclomethasone 50.
- Review in surgery before oral steroids are stopped.

**Admit**

- all children with a severe bronchospasm that does not respond immediately to treatment
- all children with a persistent bronchospasm, particularly if they are getting worse.

## 4.10 The Child with a Rash

- Vast majority are not urgent medical problems, although the sight of a rash seems to generate a disproportionate amount of alarm in some parents.
- Knowledge of current epidemics may greatly aid telephone diagnosis.
- If there is no current epidemic, most likely call is for acute urticaria.
- If child is well, it is reasonable to suggest attendance at next surgery.

**See only if**

- child is obviously toxic or unwell
- you suspect that the rash is generalised purpuric or generalised bullous in nature.

**Telephone advice**

- When no need to see
  Give caller some indication of what you think the rash might be, and reassure that it is not dangerous and does not warrant urgent treatment.

Advise attendance at next available surgery, but ask to be called if the child becomes ill or develops new symptoms.

- Before seeing the child
  *Do not put any creams on the rash until I have seen it.*

**Action when seen**

- **Assessment**

- Take history of any infectious contacts, preceding symptoms, drug ingestion, itch.
- Note distribution and nature of rash.
- Perform general examination to exclude meningism, lymphadenopathy, splenomegaly and joint swellings.

| *Type of rash* | *Likely causes and features* |
|---|---|
| Maculo-papular<br>Child not ill<br>Rash itchy | Allergy |
| Urticarial | Allergy, possibly to drugs |
| Papular urticaria<br>(very itchy) | Allergy<br>Insect bites |
| Blotchy maculo-papular<br>Child febrile | Measles (eyes very red, Koplik's spots)<br>ECHO virus may give similar rash |
| Fine macular | Rubella (cervical adenitis) |
| Generalised flush with superimposed fine punctate erythema | Scarlet fever (strawberry tongue, tonsillitis, circumoral pallor) |
| Papular, turning into vesicles | Chicken pox (comes in crops; more marked on the body than on the limbs) |
| Scattered pink macules on the body | Roseola infantum syndrome<br>(fever; rash appears as the child gets better) |
| Purpura confined to one part of the body | Traumatic<br>On face, due to vomiting or whooping cough<br>On legs, due to heavily textured tights |
| Generalised purpura | Septicaemia (child febrile)<br>Meningococcal meningitis (child toxic; may be joint or abdominal pain)<br>Thrombocytopenia (child not febrile)<br>Henoch-Schönlein (may start as urticarial rash; may be history of sore throat) |

*Continued*

| *Type of rash* | *Likely causes and features* |
|---|---|
| Bullous | Scalds (obvious history)<br>Sunburn (not so obvious history)<br>Bullous impetigo (localised patches)<br>Drug rash<br>Pemphigus |
| Localised crusts | Impetigo |
| Widespread, itchy rash<br>Scratch marks | Scabies (no history of atopy; look for burrows) |

Nappy rash is considered on p. 45.

- **Management**

| *Diagnosis* | *Management* |
|---|---|
| Allergic rash | Stop all drugs<br>Apply calamine, if available |
| Urticaria | As above<br>Prescribe antihistamines |
| Angioneurotic oedema | See p. 165 |
| Viral infections | No specific treatment necessary<br>Prescribe antibiotics only if there is secondary infection (e.g. otitis media) |
| Impetigo | If over small areas, cleanse crusts regularly and apply any mild antiseptic cream<br>If over large areas, prescribe oral antibiotics |
| Scabies | Examine the rest of the family<br>Prescribe antiscabetic treatment<br>Arrange for health visitor to supervise |
| Mechanical purpura | Explain how this arose |
| Infective purpura | **Admit** |
| Henoch-Schönlein purpura | If abdominal pain, **admit**<br>Otherwise observe and investigate |
| Thrombocytopenic or undiagnosed purpura | **Admit**—if any suspicion meningitis give parental benzylpenicillin (see p. 19) |

## 4.11 The Vomiting Child

- May be a feature of any illness or emotional upset.
- Significance depends on the seriousness of the underlying condition and whether the vomiting is severe enough to cause dehydration.
- Important to find out exactly what the caller means by vomiting. Medically, it means the forceful ejection of a considerable amount of gastric contents which usually causes some distress to the child. It is to be distinguished from posseting, the regurgitation of small amounts without distress.

- Dehydration is more likely to occur if vomiting is associated with diarrhoea.

**See unless**

- the child is posseting, not vomiting
- older child has vomited only once or twice with reasonably obvious cause (e.g. post-coughing, excitement)
- older child has vomiting associated with diarrhoea, and there is no reason to suspect that the child is becoming dehydrated

**Telephone advice**

- When no need to see
  *Give frequent small amounts of clear fluid (but not solids) for 24 hours. If vomiting persists or if other symptoms develop, the child will need to be seen.*

- Before seeing the child
  *Give the child nothing except clear fluids to drink until seen.*

**Action when seen**

- **Assessment**

- Take careful history to determine sequence of events (if there is accompanying abdominal pain, which came first?).
- Look for evidence of dehydration: dry mouth, apathy, sunken fontanelle, sunken eyes, low urine output (dry nappy), lax skin, tachypnoea.
- Look for the cause of vomiting, the diagnostic probabilities of which will vary with the age of the child.

*Remember*

- In the newborn, vomiting must be regarded as a serious symptom. It may indicate congenital bowel obstruction or infection, the source of which may not be obvious. If the vomit is bile-stained, the cause is bowel obstruction.
- The assessment of dehydration in infants is very important as it is dehydration and electrolyte imbalance which may lead to death. The degree of dehydration may be seriously underestimated if hypernatraemia exists or if the child is chubby.

- The first 3 months of life

| *Cause* | *Features* |
|---|---|
| Feeding problems | Recurrent<br>Sick after feeds, often with a belch of wind<br>Baby looks well<br>Parents often anxious with a cross baby and poor feeding techniques |
| Pyloric stenosis | Recent onset<br>Baby usually 3–6 weeks old<br>Projectile vomiting during or just after a feed<br>Cross, hungry baby |

*Continued*

| *Cause* | *Features* |
|---|---|
| | Visible peristalsis<br>Pyloric tumour may be palpable |
| Hiatus hernia | Recurrent regurgitation which is worse when the baby is being handled or is lying down flat |
| Metabolic or uraemic cause | Recurrent vomiting<br>Failure to thrive<br>May also have diarrhoea |

- Vomiting at any age

| *Cause* | *Features* |
|---|---|
| Crying | Any child may vomit after a bout of screaming<br>This may be due to physical or emotional distress |
| Cough | Bouts of coughing often make children sick<br>Consider the possibility of whooping cough |
| Infections | Almost any infection can give rise to vomiting<br>In gastroenteritis, the vomiting may start well before the diarrhoea<br>Common causes are otitis media and tonsillitis<br>Remember to look for meningitis and UTI |
| Periodic syndrome | Occurs in older children who are usually rather nervous<br>Family history of migraine<br>Recurrent<br>Vomiting in bouts |
| Intestinal obstruction | Acute onset<br>Abdominal pain<br>Look for hernias, intussusception, empty rectum |
| Poisoning | Acute onset<br>May be history of eating berries, tablets etc. |
| Intracranial space-occupying lesions | Persistent vomiting, with or without CNS signs |

**Management**

This refers to the management of vomiting per se. Any underlying cause discovered would also require appropriate management.

Parents must clearly understand that

- Vomiting, with or without diarrhoea, caused by gastroenteritis will settle on its own within 1–3 days
- Limiting intake to clear fluids only will decrease vomiting.
- Antibiotics are not necessary.
- Fluid replacement is all important and suitable clear fluids include water, flat lemonade, squash or commercially available preparations but not homemade electrolyte solutions with either added sugar or salt.

| *Assessment* | *Management* |
|---|---|
| Acute vomiting with no dehydration | Withdraw milk and solid food from the diet until the acute vomiting has abated, though breast feeding of infants should continue.<br>Give clear fluids in small volumes frequently and continue to do so no matter how many times the child vomits.<br>For infants achieve a target input of fluid for the day. (This should be worked out by the doctor on the basis of 150–200 ml per kg per 24 hours.)<br>After 24–48 hours of clear fluids milk or solids can be re-introduced.<br>Do NOT give any antiemetics. |
| Clinically detectable dehydration<br>or persistent vomiting preventing oral fluid intake<br>or the possibility of severe infection elsewhere<br>or diagnostic doubt<br>or parents not coping at home | **Admit** |
| Recurrent vomiting with no dehydration | Advise frequent small feeds of clear fluids, no solids, until the acute vomiting has settled.<br>Arrange for surgery follow up, investigation and referral as necessary. |

**Before leaving**

- allay anxiety by careful explanation to parents
- ensure that the parents know the signs of dehydration and will call again if the child worsens or does not improve in 12–24 hours
- if the cause is a virulent gastroenteritis take a faecal sample of rectal swab to see if campylobacter is the cause and therefore antibiotics indicated

## 4.12 The Child with Diarrhoea

- As a symptom, diarrhoea needs no treatment, although the underlying cause or subsequent dehydration might.
- Frequent loose stools are normal in breast-fed babies; an underfed baby may also produce loose green stools.
- An inexperienced parent may telephone when an otherwise healthy baby produces 2 or 3 loose stools. Always ask about the baby's normal feeding and bowel habits; whether the baby is still eating and drinking normally; if the baby looks well; if there are any other symptoms of illness.

**See if**

- baby has passed many loose stools
- baby appears to be unwell
- there are any associated symptoms especially abdominal pain
- there is a poor social background.

**Telephone advice**

- When no need to see
  *Let child eat if wants to but in any case increase the intake of clear fluids. Call again if the diarrhoea gets worse, if the child looks ill or if new symptoms develop.*

- Before seeing the child
  *No food, but only clear fluids until seen.*

**Action when seen**

- **Assessment**

- Look for signs of dehydration: dry mouth, dry nappy, slack skin, depressed fontanelle, drowsy apathetic behaviour.
- Look for other signs of disease, particularly otitis media and respiratory infection.

*Remember*

- Diarrhoea may be an early symptom in surgical conditions of the abdomen, so examine the abdomen carefully in every case.

- **Management**

| *Assessment* | *Management* |
|---|---|
| Baby not dehydrated and no serious underlying cause | Let child eat if wants to. Give frequent feeds of clear fluids (see management of vomiting, p. 38) If diarrhoea has persisted for more than 24–48 hours consider using Dioralyte to help replace electrolyte losses Do not prescribe antidiarrhoeal drugs |
| Baby shows evidence of dehydration or is toxic | **Admit** |

**Before leaving**

- remember that babies can deteriorate very quickly and may need to be seen again in a few hours
- ensure that the parents will call again if the child appears to worsen.

## 4.13 The Child with Abdominal Pain

- Most parents seeking an urgent consultation for a child with abdominal pain are worrying about appendicitis.
- Appendicitis must also be uppermost in your mind, as it can occur at any age and both the symptoms and signs are often atypical.
- The diagnosis can often be made from a careful history taken by telephone, but a young child with pain is likely to be frightened and a good history may not be available.
- A number of children suffer from recurrent attacks of abdominal pain. These are usually central and colicky and may be associated with vomiting. In the large majority, there is no organic cause, and anxiety in the child or parents is important aetiologically. Unfortunately, each attack presented urgently must be taken seriously. The only way to avoid missing a significant condition is by examining the child.

**See**

- unless there is only colicky pain clearly associated with diarrhoea, although if there is only a short history of colicky pain, a judicious delay may make diagnosis and assessment easier.

**Telephone advice**

- Before seeing the child
  *Do not give the child anything to eat or drink until seen.*

**Action when seen**

- **Assessment**
  - Retake history.
  - Observe the child to determine whether pain is constant or colicky.
  - Perform general examination to detect other illness (e.g. tonsillitis) which may be associated with abdominal pains.
  - Patiently examine abdomen (in younger children, may be best to keep hand gently on tummy while the baby is being cuddled by Mum).
  - Take temperature and pulse rate.
  - Check hernial orifices.
  - Check testicles.

| *Type of pain* | *Causes* | *Features* |
|---|---|---|
| Colicky pain<br>Intermittent and griping | Evening colic in babies | Commonest between 4 and 12 weeks<br>Bouts of crying<br>Feeding normally<br>Drawing up knees<br>No physical signs |
| | Gastroenteritis or bowel irritations due to upper respiratory tract infections or dietary indiscretions | Can occur at any age<br>Spasms of pain which can be sharp or griping<br>In between the spasms, abdomen soft<br>Other evidence of gastroenteritis or respiratory tract infection<br>Pain often worst just before a vomit or bowel motion |

*Continued*

| *Type of pain* | *Causes* | *Features* |
|---|---|---|
| | Intussusception | Commonest at 5–9 months<br>Severe colic<br>Child is well in between spasms, pale with them<br>May be diarrhoea in the early stages<br>Mass (sausage-shaped) may be palpable<br>PR blood, like redcurrant jelly |
| Persistent epigastric pain | Gastritis due to virus infection or tonsillitis | Some upper respiratory tract infections or attacks of epidemic vomiting may give dull epigastric pain |
| | Pneumonia | Pneumonia may give pain referred to upper abdomen<br>High temperature<br>May be painful or rapid breathing |
| | Infectious hepatitis | History of contact<br>Slow onset<br>Nausea<br>Jaundice<br>Tender Liver |
| | Mumps | Other evidence of mumps or history of contact with mumps |
| Persistent pain in the umbilical area or lower abdomen | Appendicitis | Vomiting starts after pain<br>Classically, pain is central, then moves to RIF<br>Temperature and pulse both raised<br>Tenderness and guarding in RIF<br>PR reveals tenderness to the right<br>NB: In 20% of cases, pain remains near the umbilicus |
| | Mesenteric adenitis | Obvious respiratory tract infection<br>Often high temperature<br>Tenderness less than in appendicitis<br>If in doubt, do NOT make this diagnosis; treat as appendicitis |
| | Urinary tract infection | May be symptoms such as frequency or dysuria<br>Pain not well localised<br>Look for loin tenderness<br>Dip stick test for nitrates, blood, protein |
| | Constipation | No fever<br>No guarding or significant tenderness<br>Loaded colon and rectum |
| | Strangulated hernia<br>Torsion of the testis | Severe low abdominal pain with vomiting<br>Swelling near hernial orifice or testicle<br>Remember to LOOK for this |

**● Management**

| *Assessment* | *Management* |
|---|---|
| Non-surgical cause | Do NOT use analgesics<br>Treat underlying condition |
| ANY acute surgical condition | **Admit** |
| Undiagnosed or persistent pain | **Admit** |

**Before leaving**

- ensure that the parents will call you if the pains change in character or if there is no improvement within a few hours
- arrange for follow-up, either by seeing again in a few hours time or by asking the parents to phone you with a progress report (if they forget, phone them or visit).

## 4.14 The Acutely Constipated Child

- May present as a 'screamer'.
- Often secondary to recurrent constipation associated with behaviour problems.
- Crisis caused by large lump of faeces which produces pain when the child tries to expel it.

**● Telephone advice**

- When no need to see
  Reassure the parents that this is not serious. Advise them to insert some Vaseline into the rectum by finger or to use a glycerine suppository, if they have one. If they do not succeed, the child will need to be seen, as it may scream for some time.

**Action when seen**

**● Assessment**

- Examine the abdomen and perform PR.

**● Management**

- Try to break up the hard mass of faeces with a gloved finger covered with plenty of KY jelly, and remove the faeces bit by bit.

**Before leaving**

- advise the parents to use a mixture of firmness and encouragement, a high-fibre diet and judicious use of glycerine suppositories to ensure that the child's bowels open regularly
- mention that you will be asking the health visitor to supervise progress.

## 4.15 Rectal Prolapse

- Rectal mucosa may prolapse in small, normal children.
- Very alarming for parents, who will telephone saying 'his bowel is dropping out'.

- Self-limiting condition, occasionally associated with fibrocystic disease or meningomyelocoele.

**See if**

- this is the first episode.

**Action when seen**

- **Management**
  - Elevate the child's buttocks.
  - Using a glove and plenty of KY jelly, ease the mucosa back into the rectum with the flat of the finger.
  - Teach the parents how to do this, as the condition will almost certainly recur.

## 4.16 The Fitting Child

- One in twelve children will have had a fit of some sort by the age of 11 years.
- Small babies tend not to have a classical tonic or clonic fit, but to choke, go blue, jerk or go stiff.
- Most likely to be febrile fit, but if recurrent may be epilepsy.
- In babies, may be caused by birth injury, hypoglycaemia, hypocalcaemia or infection.
- Meningitis must always be excluded.
- Caller is usually very upset and is often afraid that the child is dying.

**Visit**

**Telephone advice**

- When about to visit
  *I am coming. While I am on my way, you must keep calm. If the child has vomited, clean out his mouth so that he does not choke, then lie him on his side. If the child is very hot, take his clothes off and sponge the head and body with lukewarm water.*

**Action when seen**

- **Assessment**
  - If the child is still fitting, proceed directly to Management.
  - If the episode is over, ascertain whether it was a fit, faint or breath-holding attack.

| | *Faint* | *Breath-holding attack* | *Fit* |
|---|---|---|---|
| *Age* | Older child | Toddler | Any age |
| *Onset* | Gradual | Preceded by screaming | No warning |
| *Precipitating factors* | Warmth, change of posture, emotion | Temper, frustration | Usually none<br>If a febrile fit, fever |
| *Colour* | White | Blue | May be blue during the tonic phase |
| *After the attack* | Quick recovery | Quick recovery | Dazed<br>May go to sleep |

- If you think that it was a fit, take a detailed history to discover if there has been any history of fits, if there is any relevant family history and if there has been any preceding illness, trauma or fever.
- Examine the child, paying particular attention to the state of arousal, the CNS and finding the cause of any fever.

**• Management**

| *Assessment* | *Management* |
|---|---|
| Fit still in progress | Stesolid 5 mg rectal tube: 1–3 years one tube inserted halfway to mark on nozzle; 4 years or more – two tubes. In both cases if no effect is seen after 5 minutes the same dose may be given again. **or** If an older child and it is easy to get into a vein, give diazepam (0.15–0.25 mg per kg body weight) SLOW IV, until eyelids droop or fitting stops **Admit** |
| Fit stopped | |
| First fit | **Admit** |
| Recurrent fit | If you have any suspicion that this fit has been caused by meningitis, **admit,** after giving parenteral benzylpenicillin (see p. 19) If the fit is exactly as before and there are no sequelae, keep at home |
| Recurrent febrile fit | If you have any suspicion that this fit has been caused by meningitis, **admit,** after giving parenteral benzylpenicillin (see p. 19) otherwise paracetamol every 4 hours Fanning or tepid sponging If there is a risk or recurrence, give rectal diazepam in the dose shown above Antibiotics, if indicated, to treat the cause of the fever. |

**Before leaving**

- arrange to see the child again in a few hours
- arrange to review the long-term management, if the fits are recurrent.

## 4.17 Acute Genitourinary Problems

- Most likely presentation is because of pain or difficulty in passing urine.
- Obtaining a good history by telephone may allow diagnosis to be made and advice to be given.

| *Diagnosis* | *Features* | *Management* |
|---|---|---|
| Urinary tract infection (see p. 177) | Frequency<br>Dysuria<br>Fever<br>May present as PUO or abdominal pain | If child is feverish and toxic, see soon<br>If child is not ill, see later in the surgery<br>Obtain MSU specimen or dipslide before treatment<br>Increase fluid intake<br>Commence Amoxil or Trimethoprim course<br>Follow-up is essential to decide whether further investigation is necessary |
| Dysuria or nappy rash | Dysuria may be from UTI, but more frequently is from ammonia dermatitis of the vulva or foreskin<br>May be a lot of pain, so a visit is demanded | Advise as for nappy rash:<br>Keep nappy off for 24 hours<br>Apply any bland cream frequently<br>Maintain a high fluid intake<br>Arrange for follow-up by health visitor<br>If child needs to be seen, immediate relief will be given if the sore area is wiped with cotton wool moistened with lignocaine 1% |
| Retention of urine | Newborn babies may not pass urine until 12 hours after birth<br>In older children, usually voluntary because of scalding | If true retention, **admit** |
| Scrotal swelling (see p. 176) | When noticed, the parent may panic and seek advice<br>If painful, regard as torsion of the testicle until proved otherwise<br>If swelling extends into inguinal canal, this may rarely be from an incarcerated hernia | If painless, see at next surgery<br>If painful, see quickly<br>Torsion of the testicle, **admit**<br>Incarcerated hernia, **admit** |

*Continued*

| Diagnosis | Features | Management |
|---|---|---|
| Haematuria (see p. 172) | Must be taken seriously<br>Remember—urine can be coloured by blackcurrant juice or beetroot | If child is not ill and there are no other symptoms, see quickly<br>Test urine with Multistix<br>If bleeding is mild, advise high fluid intake and investigate<br>If bleeding is moderate or continuous, **admit** |

For balanitis, see p. 172.
For paraphimosis, see. p. 173.
For testicular pain, see p. 175.

## 4.18 The Child with a Limp or Pain in the Limbs

- A limp or complaint that a child will not use its arm is a fairly common cause of an emergency call.

**Direct to A & E if**
- there is a history of major trauma

Otherwise,

**See child urgently**

**Action when seen**

- **Assessment**
  - Take plenty of time to observe the child's movements and walking.
  - Undress the child completely and examine carefully for localised tenderness, bruising and joint mobility.
  - Consider the possibility of child abuse.

| *Diagnosis* | *Features* | *Management* |
|---|---|---|
| Fracture | Local tenderness<br>No fever<br>Little swelling at first<br>NB: Do not forget clavicle or greensticks | **Refer** to A & E |
| Osteomyelitis | Pain<br>Tenderness<br>Swelling<br>Fever (progressive) | **Admit** |
| Pulled elbow | Complaint that child 'will not use arm'<br>Occurs mainly in 1–4 year olds | Manipulate:<br>Hold the lower end of the humerus with the left hand |

*Continued*

| *Diagnosis* | *Features* | *Management* |
|---|---|---|
| | Story of falling while being held by the hand or of being pulled up by the hand<br>Pain on moving the elbow | Taking the wrist in the right hand, smoothly turn the forearm into full supination |
| Transient synovitis of the hip | Occurs mainly in 2–6 year olds<br>No fever or toxic symptoms<br>No inflamed muscles or glands<br>Limited hip movements | Advise strict rest<br>Analgesia as required<br>Follow-up in 24 hours<br>Arrange for FBC and X-ray of hips, if necessary<br>If severe, **admit,** as it is not possible to exclude infection |
| Painful hip in older child | In 5–10 year old, likely to be Perthes' disease<br>In 10–15 year old, likely to be slipped epiphysis<br>**Remember**—hip disease may present as pain in the knee | As for transient synovitis of the hip |
| Night pains | Severe pains in the legs of young children<br>May cause screaming attacks<br>Bilateral | If bilateral, starts after child has gone to bed, no fever or other toxic symptoms, advise simple analgesics |

## 4.19 The Child Who Has Swallowed Something

- An infinite variety of small objects, vegetable matter, medicines and household products may be involved.
- Once discovered, panic and guilt will lead to an urgent call for advice.
- Decision to make is whether child can be kept at home and observed, or whether child must be taken to A & E for possible X-ray, specific antidote or admission.
- In all cases, primary concern is support of vital functions, not elimination of poison.
- National Poisons Information Service (see p. 49 for telephone number) may be able to provide useful information and advice.
- Do not use emetics as are of very limited value.
- In some cases activated charcoal may be useful first line support. May be effective up to 2 hours or more after ingestion. For children dose is 1g/kg (available as liquid).

● **Management**

| | |
|---|---|
| ● Small objects | ANY suspicion that an object has been inhaled rather than ingested, **refer** to A & E<br>ANY object with sharp or pointed edges, or a shape that may impede its transmission through the bowel, **refer** to A & E<br>Other objects can be left to pass naturally, but instruct parents to call again if any symptoms develop |
| ● Plants and fungi | Fear of poisoning is more imagined than real<br>If you have identified the plant, guidance of National Poisons Information Service may be sought<br>If plant is unknown, advise parents to take a sample and the child to A & E |
| ● Drugs and medicines | Medicine is usually known, but generally the amount is not<br>In cases where you are not sure of likely effect or danger, seek guidance of Poisons Information Services<br>Patients who have taken poisons with delayed actions should be refered to A & E even if they appear well. Delayed action poisons include aspirin, iron, paracetamol, tricyclic antidepressants, Lomotil, and modified release capsules<br>ANY likely toxicity, **refer** to A & E |
| ● Household products | Vast majority are not hazardous when swallowed in small quantities<br>Liquids and pellets are most likely to be ingested in large quantities, especially if they have a nice flavour<br>Many products (e.g. bleach) are much more hazardous if taken in large quantities<br>Kettle descalers, drain cleaners, dishwashing machine powders, battery acid are dangerous whatever quantity ingested as is any petroleum distillate e.g. turps.<br>In all cases advise parents not to try to make child sick or to give them salt and water or milk. Just give a small glass of water, ensure child is warm and not in shock. For skin contact wash with water, preferably with a few drops of detergent. For chemicals is the eye an eyewash at home is advisable before attending hospital.<br>Try to determine quantity (from parents) and toxicity (from Poisons Information Service) before deciding whether to observe at home or **refer** to A & E (get parents to take substance with them) |

## POISONS INFORMATION CENTRES (consult day and night)

| | | |
|---|---|---|
| Belfast | | (01232) 240503 |
| Birmingham | | 0121-507 5588 |
| | *or* | 0121-507 5589 |
| Cardiff | | (01222) 709901 |
| Dublin | | Dublin 837 9964 |
| | *or* | Dublin 837 9966 |
| Edinburgh | | 0131-536 2300 |
| Leeds | | (0113) 243 0715 |
| | *or* | (0113) 292 3547 |
| London | | 0171-635 9191 |
| | *or* | 0171-955 5095 |
| Newcastle | | 0191-232 5131 |

*Note.* Some of these centres also advise on laboratory analytical services which may be of help in the diagnosis and management of a small number of cases

Do not give phone number to patients
When call have following information available

—name and amount of substance swallowed
—time since exposure
—name, age, weight (in kg) of patient

**Notes**

# 5 Cardiovascular Emergencies

*Disorders of the cardiovascular system provide some of the more dramatic emergencies that the GP has to face. This chapter aims to provide a working guide to the primary care of such emergencies. For this reason, the differential diagnosis of presenting symptoms is only explored as far as is necessary for immediate management. The rarer disorders have not been mentioned, because detailed investigation is not practical in a general practice emergency.*

## Chapter Contents



See also Differential diagnosis of acute breathlessness, p. 158

# 5.1 Chest Pain

- Cause of great anxiety both to patient and those in attendance, hence a common reason for an emergency call.
- Minor musculoskeletal and anxiety pains are common, but usually present in surgery.
- Details of site, duration, radiation, character, associated symptoms and previous episodes are necessary, and may be gained over the phone while deciding whether to visit. If pain is severe or anxiety great, the caller may resist questioning, and details must be left until visit.

**Dial 999 for ambulance**

- If from description you are reasonably sure patient is having a myocardial infarction.
- Advise relatives to get patient to chew 300 mg aspirin while waiting (can be as effective as thrombolytic therapy in reducing mortality).
- Visit as well if you are likely to arrive significantly before the ambulance—advise patient not to wait for you if ambulance arrives first.

**See**

- Unless the cause is obviously oesophagitis, tracheitis or musculoskeletal
- If in any doubt about the diagnosis

**Telephone advice**

- Before seeing

  *Keep the patient comfortable until seen.*

**General assessment**

- If the patient is pale, sweaty, fearful and holding the centre of the chest, a spot diagnosis of ischaemic heart pain may be made.
- Otherwise, a detailed history and careful examinataion are needed before diagnosing.
- Chest pain resulting from cardiovascular causes may be accompanied by some clinical signs of cardiac distress (e.g. tachycardia, poor cardiac output, soft first sound, dysrhythmias, pulmonary oedema, raised venous pressure and breathlessness).
- Unfortunately abnormal signs are often absent and diagnosis may have to be based on history alone.
- ECG is very useful diagnostically, but only if you are sure that you can interpret the traces competently.

## 5.1.1 Differential Diagnosis

| *Pain* | *Likely diagnosis* | *Special features* |
|---|---|---|
| Retrosternal, radiating across chest and possibly into arms and neck | Myocardial ischaemia or infarction | Pain may be poorly localised, and described as tight or constricting<br>Severe apprehension common<br>If pain lasts more than 20 minutes, infarction indicated rather than ischaemia |

*Continued*

| *Pain* | *Likely diagnosis* | *Special features* |
|---|---|---|
| | Hiatus hernia or oesophagitis | Often burning pain which is worse after food, on stooping or lying down<br>Discomfort worst at lower end of sternum |
| As above, but going into or starting in back | Dissecting aneurysm | Severe tearing pain<br>Pulses in neck or limb may be absent |
| | Posterior infarction | May be other evidence of cardiac damage |
| Central and persistent, which may vary with respiration and be reduced on leaning forward | Pericarditis | Friction rub<br>May be signs of systemic viral infection<br>Effusion may give dull pain with evidence of tamponade |
| 'Raw' and central, which is worse on coughing | Tracheitis | Signs and symptoms of respiratory infection |
| Lateral chest, which is worse on respiration | Pleurisy | Pleural rub<br>Evidence of pneumonia |
| | Pneumothorax | Sudden onset<br>Poor air entry<br>Hyperresonance |
| | Pulmonary infarction | Haemoptysis<br>Tachypnoea<br>Tachycardia<br>Possible DVT |
| | Bornholm's | Pain poorly localised<br>Fever<br>Tender muscles |
| | Trauma<br>Cough fracture<br>Costochondritis<br>Secondaries | History<br>Tender to touch |
| | Diaphragmatic catch syndrome | No trauma<br>Transient pain which 'catches the breath'<br>Tender rib margins |
| Radiating in a band around the chest | Nerve root pressure | Pain worsened by moving spine or pressure on spine |
| | Herpes zoster | Pain and hyperaesthesia may precede rash by several days |

If any moderate or severe pain in the chest, arms, neck, face or upper abdomen is unexplained or associated with any cardiac symptoms, consider myocardial infarction as a diagnosis.

- Remember an infarct may be painless, especially in the elderly.

## 5.1.2 Myocardial Ischaemia and Myocardial Infarction

**Action when seen**

- **Assessment**

| *Pain* | *Diagnosis* |
|---|---|
| Of short duration, particularly if there is a history of angina | Probably due to ischaemia rather than infarction |
| Of more than 20 minutes duration or which persists despite glyceryl trinitrite or sorbitrate | Should be regarded as myocardial infarction |

- **Management**

| | |
|---|---|
| Myocardial ischaemia | Nitrolingual spray 2–4 puffs sublingually. If relief not rapid then treat as myocardial infarction. |
| Myocardial infarction | Treat pain:<br>Cyclimorph (10 mg) IV slowly; if insufficient, give further 5–10 mg in 15 minutes<br>Treat arrhythmias:<br>Atropine (0.6 mg) slow IV for bradycardia (pulse less than 50) **or** lignocaine (100 mg) slow IV for multiple ectopic beats (10 ml of 1% solution)<br>Treat failure:<br>If breathless with creps. at bases, frusemide (40 mg) IV<br>Treat thrombus:<br>Get patient to chew sol. aspirin 300 mg or use clotbuster, if available, as per local protocol |

**You must admit unless**

- the patient wants to stay at home after the pros and cons have been explained AND
- there is good pain relief and patient is in good general condition
- more than 24 hours have elapsed since the onset of the symptoms
- the home conditions and communications are good.

**Before leaving**

When **admission** necessary:

- ensure the patient travels in an ambulance with oxygen
- ask for patient to arrange to see you after discharge from hospital.

If home care being provided:

- arrange to revisit in 4 hours
- arrange for ECG and assay of cardiac enzymes, to confirm diagnosis and assess severity of infarct
- ensure that those in attendance realise that there is a risk involved in home care, although admission to hospital does not necessarily lower the risk.

## 5.1.3 Cardiac Arrest

**Action when seen**

- **Assessment**
  - Unlikely to be treated successfully in general practice.
  - Irreversible brain damage occurs within 3–4 minutes of cessation of cerebral circulation; if you were not present at time of arrest, probably best to certify death.
  - If patient is youngish and you and relatives were present when the arrest occurred, it may be worthwhile attempting cardiopulmonary resuscitation.

- **Management**
  - Tell someone to dial 999 for an ambulance.
  - Put patient onto firm surface.
  - Give firm blow to lower sternum with side of closed fist.
  - Compress lower third of sternum with heel of one hand, with other hand on top, and elbow extended so that full body weight used.
  - Compress at rate of about 60 per minute, displacing sternum 4–5 cm with each compression.
  - Give 4 or 5 compressions for each lung inflation.
  - If possible, get someone to use the airway to respirate the patient or to perform mouth-to-mouth resuscitation: otherwise, do it yourself:

    pinch the patient's nose
    fully extend his head
    hold his jaw forward
    place your mouth in contact with his and blow remove your mouth and allow the patient to exhale passively.
    NB: One person cannot keep this up for long. If there is no sign of an ambulance and/or no sign of recovery in the patient (pupils fixed and dilated), stop and admit that the patient is dead.
  - Use defibrillator, if available, as per local protocol.

### 5.1.4 Other Causes of Chest Pain

**Action when seen**

- **Management**

| *Diagnosis* | *Management* |
|---|---|
| Suspected embolism | **Admit** in ambulance with oxygen |
| Dissecting aneurysm | As for myocardial infarction: **admit** |
| Pericarditis | As for myocardial infarction: **admit** |
| Pleurisy | See pneumonia (p. 163) |
| Pneumothorax | See pneumothorax (p. 166) |
| Oesophagitis | Antacids<br>Advice |
| Tracheitis | Hot drinks and analgesia |
| Nerve root pressure; Herpes zoster; Bornholm's; trauma; cough fracture; secondaries; costochondritis | Appropriate analgesia<br>Advice<br>Follow-up and investigation |
| Diaphragmatic catch | Reassurance |

## 5.2 Heart Failure

### 5.2.1 Acute Left Ventricular Failure

- Common cause of emergency calls, especially during the night.
- Generally presents with sudden-onset dyspnoea, severe distress and possible production of frothy, blood-stained sputum.
- May present insidiously, with complaint of persistent cough accompanied by some breathlessness or wheezing: beware of out-of-hours call to older patient with 'another attack of bronchitis'.
- Generally, an elder panicky caller who will not tolerate much telephone questioning.

**Visit**

**Telephone advice**

- When about to visit
  *Prop the patient up. I will be with you as soon as possible.*

**Action when seen**

- **Assessment**

- Diagnosis usually obvious.
- Do not waste time on detailed history or examination.
- If bases are wet and patient is distressed, start treatment.
- If any doubt whether asthma or bronchitis, see Table on p. 160.

| | |
|---|---|
| ● **Management** | ● Cyclimorph (10 mg IV slowly; less for very old patient) (N.B. ONLY if in no doubt about diagnosis.)<br>● Frusemide (40 mg) IV.<br>● If no better in 10–15 minutes Nitrolingual spray 2 puffs sublingually<br>● Oxygen, if available. |

**Admit if**

- there is not a good response to treatment
- you cannot ensure proper nursing and monitoring of patient for the next few hours
- underlying pathology needs urgent treatment (e.g. onset of fibrillation in mitral stenosis).

**Before leaving**

- appreciate that if the patient stays at home, you will need to revisit within 4 hours
- decide about long-term diuretic therapy and ACE inhibitors
- assess the need for treatment of any underlying pathology including hypertension and whether referral or other investigation such as echocardiogram is needed.

## 5.2.2 Congestive Heart Failure

- Characterised by dependent oedema, enlarged liver and elevated JVP.
- Usually slow in onset, with presentation in surgery because of oedema or progressive dyspnoea.
- Elderly patients may neglect to call you until symptoms become very severe and require an emergency visit.

**Visit**

**Telephone advice**

- When about to visit
  *Tell patient to sit and rest until I arrive.*

**Action when seen**

● **Assessment**

- Assess degree of failure.
- Assess general condition of patient.
- Examine for any underlying pathology (e.g. anaemia, arrhythmias, valvular lesions).

| | |
|---|---|
| ● **Management** | ● Frusemide (80 mg) oral. |

**Admit if**

- oedema is very severe (marked diuresis may produce profound electrolyte disturbances or acute retention)
- Patient lives in poor social conditions.

**Before leaving**

- ensure that it is understood that regular checks will be necessary until the patient is mobile and the heart failure controlled
- arrange to see patient again within 12 hours to assess progress, adjust diuretic therapy, consider digitilization or ACE inhibition and check serum electrolytes.

## 5.3 Arrhythmias

- Sudden changes in cardiac rhythm may cause very unpleasant sensations or precipitate changes in consciousness.
- Once the patient has noticed a change in heart rhythm, the understandable worry that something serious is amiss may lead to an urgent consultation being sought.
- Symptoms such as the heart missing a beat, racing, beating irregularly or having palpitations need careful consideration.

**See unless**

- symptoms are transient and patient has no history of heart disease
- patient accepts reassurance and is willing to wait for a routine appointment.

**Telephone advice**

- Before seeing
  *Do not worry; this is unlikely to be serious. Keep the patient calm until seen.*

**Action when seen**

- **Assessment**
  - Unless the patient is seen during an attack, the diagnosis of a transient arrhythmia depends on a careful history and examination to detect any underlying heart disease.
  - Persistent arrhythmia is best diagnosed definitively with an ECG, although the clinically-based table below allows for formulation of a safe plan of immediate management.

| *Symptoms* | *Causes* | *Features* |
|---|---|---|
| Irregular heart beats<br>Heart misses a beat<br>Heart thumps | Ectopic beats (supraventricular, nodal or ventricular) | Irregular pulse<br>Usually normal rate<br>Pulse more regular on exercise or with anxiety<br>Patient either notices a missed beat or the following strong beat felt as a thump |
| | Slow atrial fibrillation | Irregular pulse. Does not become more regular with exercise |
| Palpitations<br>Heart racing | Ordinary sinus tachycardia | Rate usually 120 or less, and changes gradually<br>Associated with anxiety, thyrotoxicosis or other systemic disturbance |
| | Paroxysmal tachycardias (supraventricular or nodal) | Rate 160 or more, regular, fixed<br>Changes in rate are sudden<br>Often responds to vagal stimulation (Valsalva)<br>Not usually associated with other heart disease |
| | Paroxysmal ventricular tachycardia | Rate 160 or more, regular, fixed<br>Changes in rate are sudden |

*Continued*

| *Symptoms* | *Causes* | *Features* |
|---|---|---|
| | | Does not respond to vagal stimulation (Valsalva)<br>Often associated with other heart disease |
| | Atrial flutter | Rate about 100–150, fixed<br>May occasionally be 250 or more<br>Vagal stimulation (e.g. Valsalva) changes rate suddenly, but it reverts when this stops |
| | Paroxysmal atrial fibrillation | Fast, irregular pulse |
| Syncope<br>Feeling faint<br>Blackouts | Paroxysmal tachycardias | As above<br>Sudden fast heart rates may induce faintness |
| | Heart block | Slow pulse<br>50 or below usually indicates heart block<br>40 or below usually causes syncope<br>Heart sounds vary in loudness |
| Breathlessness | Any dysrhythmia causing large changes in heart rates may produce a drop in cardiac output | Sudden changes of rhythm will cause acute dyspnoea<br>Long-standing dysrhythmias will produce slowly progressive dyspnoea and signs of congestive cardiac failure |

● **Management**

The correct diagnosis may be suspected on clinical grounds, but can only be positively made after ECG. Our management assumes that no ECG is immediately available and that some diagnoses can be made with reasonable certainty on clinical grounds alone.

| *Diagnosis* | *Management* |
|---|---|
| ANY arrhythmia associated with acute myocardial ischaemia | **Admit** |
| Extrasystoles | No immediate treatment necessary<br>NB: May be a sign of digoxin toxicity |
| Sinus tachycardia | No immediate treatment necessary |
| Paroxysmal tachycardia | Try vagal stimulation (perform Valsalva manoeuvre or make patient gag by putting fingers down throat) |

*Continued*

| *Diagnosis* | *Management* |
|---|---|
| | If this fails, try unilateral carotid sinus pressure, using three fingers pressed on the carotid artery at the level of the thyroid cartilage<br>NB: Not if carotid bruit<br>Take care in elderly<br>Success implies paroxysmal supraventricular tachycardia: prescribe beta-blocker<br>Failure: **admit** |
| Fibrillation | If of recent onset, admit for rhythm correction<br>In an elderly patient, if you wish to control the heart rate but not correct the rhythm, digitalise at home using Digoxin (0.5 mg) oral stat., then 0.25 mg daily until controlled. Start soluble aspirin 150 mg daily unless contradicated. |
| ANY arrhythmia causing changes of consciousness | **Admit** or refer urgently |

**Before leaving**

- remember that, except for cases with occasional ectopics and no evidence of heart disease, the patient will need ECG and investigation for any underlying cause, e.g. thyrotoxicosis.
- consider in fibrillating patients whether they should be anticoagulated or not.

## 5.4 Hypertension

- Presents as an emergency when a complication arises (e.g. CVA, acute LVF, rapid loss of vision).
- In most cases, it is the presenting problem which requires treatment, and hypotensive therapy may be instituted routinely.
- Headache or rapid blurring of vision, associated with papilloedema and increased blood pressure, idicate malignant hypertension. If this is suspected, urgent **admission** is indicated.

## 5.5 Temporal Arteritis

- Disease of late middle age and old age, which may present with polymyalgia or as headache.
- Diagnosed by acute tenderness along course of temporal or occipital arteries.

- Can cause sudden blindness if retinal arteries are involved.
- Do not dismiss request for urgent consultation for headache, especially if headache is severe or persistent in someone who does not usually suffer from them.

**See**

**Action when seen**

- **Management**
  - Take blood for ESR as soon as possible, but do not wait for results before starting treatment (a high ESR confirms the diagnosis, and referral and/or long-term follow-up will be required).
  - Prednisolone (30 mg) stat. followed by a course gradually reducing the minimum effective maintenance level.

## 5.6 Acute Arterial Insufficiency of the Limbs

- Generally affects legs rather than arms.
- In patients with generalised arteriosclerosis, is caused by sudden embolic or thrombotic obstruction.
- Possibly no history of peripheral ischaemia, but may be some history of cardiac disease.
- Very acute pain reaching a maximum within minutes, although occasionally it may build up over hours.
- Frequently associated with sensations of numbness, coldness, tingling and weakness.

**Visit**

**Telephone advice**
- Before seeing
  *Keep the limb down and do not warm it. I will be with you as quickly as I can.*

**Action when seen**

- **Assessment**
  - Patient usually very distressed.
  - Limb initially pale, then takes on mottled and/or cyanotic colour.
  - Try to determine level of obstruction by feeling for peripheral pulses and temperature change on skin.
- **Management**
  - Cyclimorph (15 mg) IM.
  - **ADMIT** preferably to a hospital with a vascular surgeon.
  - Do NOT warm the limb.

## 5.7 Acute Venous Problems

### 5.7.1 Superficial Thrombophlebitis

- Not a serious problem, but patients may seek urgent consultation because of general fear of 'thrombosis'.
- If clearly only superficial tenderness, patient may be seen routinely, although patient may need to be seen quickly if anxiety is great.

**Telephone advice**
- When not necessary to see
  *This does not cause clots in the lungs. Take soluble aspirin every 4 hours. Make a routine appointment.*

## 5.7.2 Deep Vein Thrombosis

- A painful or swollen calf, particularly in a woman taking the contraceptive pill, is the usual reason for an emergency call.
- Half the cases are asymptomatic and may present as pulmonary embolism.
- When confined to the calf, extremely unlikely to give rise to emboli.
- If calf symptoms are sudden in onset, they are more likely to be caused by a muscle tear or haemorrhage than by a DVT.

**See**

**Telephone advice**
- Before seeing
  *Put your feet up and take 2 aspirins. I will see you later.*

**Action when seen**

- **Assessment**
  - Painful, tender and swollen calf.
  - Pain exacerbated by dorsiflexion of foot.
- **Management**
  - Urgent **referral** to hospital for anticoagulation

## 5.7.3 Bleeding Varicose Vein

- Story of severe bleeding from lower limb without major trauma is almost certain to be due to a burst varicose vein.

**Urgent visit if**
- patient is alone
- caller is too panicky to perform first aid
- bleeding does not stop, or recurs after first aid.

**Telephone advice**
- When about to visit
  *Calm down; this can be dealt with easily. Lie the patient down, and raise the leg above the level of the body. Get someone to press on the bleeding point with a pad. I shall be with you shortly.*

**Action when seen**

- **Assessment**
  - Patient's general condition is related to the amount of blood apparently lost.
  - Have the first aid measures been effective?
- **Management**
  - Firmly bandage with whatever bandages are available.
  - Prescribe crepe bandages and non-stick dressings (to be applied later by district nurse).
  - If blood loss severe or patient shocked, **admit**.

**Before leaving**
- ask patient to attend surgery routinely later.

# 6 Dermatological Emergencies

*It is rare for an urgent visit to be requested for an adult with a skin disorder. However, telephone advice may well be sought.*

## Chapter Contents

## 6.1 Animal Bites and Scratches

- The risks to consider are those of tetanus and wound infection.
- Remember that tetanus toxoid is a long term preventative measure; if a real risk of tetanus exists, penicillin is indicated.
- If bite was sustained abroad, consider the possibility of rabies developing.

**Telephone advice**

- When no need to see
  Skin not broken, or superficial scratch or graze
  *Clean with an antiseptic. Is a tetanus booster needed?*

  Skin broken
  *Clean the wound thoroughly with water and antiseptic. Patient will require a tetanus booster if none given within the last year. If the wound is deep or extensive, take the patient to A & E or bring to Surgery.* Patient will need penicillin.

## 6.2 Bee and Wasp Stings

- Lethal dose for an unsensitised human is usually hundreds of stings.
- 0.5% of the population are hypersensitive to bee or wasp stings and could be killed by a single sting.
- Bee leaves a barbed sting embedded in the skin, whereas the wasp does not.

**Telephone advice**

- When no need to see
  Unsensitised patient
  *Using a blade or finger nail scrape the sting out.*
  *Clean the sting area with antiseptic. Give the patient soluble aspirin.*

  Sensitised patient
  Advise as for angioneurotic oedema (p. 165).
  *('Go to nearest medical care at once.')*

## 6.3 Burns and Scalds

- Caused by heat, electricity or chemicals.
- Superficial burns are painful, red and blistered.
- Deep burns are painless, white or brown and may be charred.
- Severity depends on depth of burn, area burnt and age of patient.

**Visit if**

- major analgesia is necessary before patient can be transported to hospital.

**Telephone advice**

- When no need to see or before seen
  Minor burn

*Hold the burnt area under cold running water or immerse it in cold water or constantly splash the face for at least 10 minutes. Do NOT attempt to remove burnt clothing from the damaged area. Do Not prick blisters or apply ointments. Cover the burnt area with some clean material. Tell patient if he or she needs help, to go to A & E/Surgery for dressings.*

Major burn

Thermal

*Smother flames. Extinguish smouldering clothing with water. Cool burnt tissue with cold water. After dowsing with cold water, remove clothing that has been saturated with hot liquids, but NOT burnt clothing adhering to the skin.*

Chemical

*Wash the corrosive off with copious amounts of water (e.g. with a fire hose).*

In both cases

- irrigate the eyes, if they were involved.
- dial 999 for an ambulance.
- wrap patient in a clean sheet.
- **admit** to A & E.

**Action when seen**

| *Assessment* | *Management* |
|---|---|
| • Minor burn | Only small, superficial burns in non-vital places should be treated at home<br>Use non-adherent dressings or leave burn exposed<br>Avoid using local antibiotics<br>Use systematic antibiotics only if burn infected<br>**Refer** all other burns to A & E |
| • Major burn | Cyclimorph IV<br>Maintain airway<br>Wrap patient in a clean sheet for transport to A & E<br>Give IV infusion, if available |

## 6.4 Lacerations

- Most patients with lacerations will be taken direct to A & E.

**Visit if**

- patient is old or lacks transport to go to A & E or come to surgery, and must be sutured at home.

**Telephone advice**

- When visit not necessary
  *Apply pressure to the bleeding part using a clean cloth. Take patient to A & E, or bring the patient to the surgery for stitching.*

## 6.5 Rashes

- Question caller carefully before dismissing the need for patient to be seen.
- Acute urticaria is the most likely reason for a call.
- For differential diagnosis of rash, see p. 34.

**See if**

- patient is suffering from major urticaria with a risk of angioneurotic oedema (see p. 165) or if appears to have a purpuric rash or if is obviously toxic.

**Telephone advice**

- When no need to see
- If you know likely diagnosis

  *Tell patient likely diagnosis.*
- If there is no obvious diagnosis

  *This is not serious, so we can wait and see what happens. Use calamine lotion or take any available antihistamine to soothe the itch. Make a routine surgery appointment. Call back if any new symptoms develop.*

## 6.6 Snake Bites

- Rare in UK, where the only poisonous snake is the adder (viper).
- In its early stages, snake bite is very unpredictable, and all victims should be kept under close hospital observation for at least 24 hours.
- If venom has been injected from an adder bite, local swelling usually starts within a few minutes though maybe up to 2 hours. This is a very valuable clinical sign; the absence of swelling indicates that envenoming can be excluded.

**See**

- Only if patient cannot be transferred to hospital as quickly as possible avoiding active movements especially of the affected limb.

**Action if seen**

- **Management**

Remain calm, avoiding active movements.
Adequately reassure patient.
If signs of early anaphylactic reaction give adrenaline (epinephrine) 0.5 ml of 0.1%, 1 in 1000 IM in adults (0.01 ml/kg in children) repeated after 5 minutes if reaction not controlled (see p. 166).
**Admit.**

## 6.7 Sunburn

- Call for advice may be for sunburn or for sunstroke.
- The delayed erythema of sunburn begins 2–4 hours after exposure and reaches a peak in 15 hours. If erythema is severe then it will be painful and uncomfortable and occasionally may blister.

- Sunstroke, if severe, presents with hyperpyrexia, nausea and weakness.

**See if**

- a child has extensive sunburn.
- history suggest sunstroke.

**Telephone advice**

- When no need to see
  *Avoid further exposure to sunlight until the redness fades. Take a cold shower or bath regularly and apply calamine lotion liberally. If necessary, take aspirin or paracetamol for the pain. Take plenty of clear, cold fluids to drink.*
- Before seeing
  *Keep as cool as you can until seen.*

**Action when seen**

| *Diagnosis* | *Management* |
|---|---|
| Sunburn | Advice as per telephone advice.<br>Prescribe a strong topical steroid cream to be applied TID for 3 days.<br>If blisters present, protect them from abrasion. |
| Sunstroke | If mild, treat associated sunburn and advise iced drinks frequently in small quantities to replace lost fluid.<br>If toxaemia, fever, nausea and weakness present then admit for IV fluids and energetic cooling. |

## 6.8 Superglue Accidents

- Superglue causes no permanent damage to skin, mucous membranes or eyes.
- Accidents are best handled by passive, non-surgical first aid.

**Telephone advice**

- When no need to see or before seen
  Skin adhesion
  *Immerse bonded surfaces in warm soapy water for 10 minutes, then peel or roll the surfaces apart with a blunt-edged instrument. Remove the adhesive using soapy water, but do NOT pull the surfaces apart with a direct opposing action. If the lips are stuck together, bathe them with plenty of warm water and press with saliva from behind. Once adequately wetted, the lips can be peeled or rolled apart, but do NOT try to pull them apart.*

  Adhesive in the eye
  *If eyelid-to-eyelid or eyelid-to-eyeball, wash thoroughly only with warm water and cover with a dry gauze pad. The eye will open within 4 days and there should be no residual damage. If there is gross contamination, however, best to go to A & E or eye unit.*

## Notes

# 7 Endocrine Emergencies

*Apart from those caused by diabetes, emergencies involving the endocrine system are rare in general practice. This chapter is therefore chiefly concerned with the management of diabetes.*

## Chapter Contents

# 7.1 Adrenocortical Insufficiency

- May be primary (Addison's disease), secondary to pituitary failure, or the result of adrenal suppression due to steroid therapy.
- Emergency presentation of new cases is extremely rare, and crises are most likely to arise in patients who have Addison's disease and are on replacement therapy, or in patients receiving, or just having completed, steroid therapy.
- Symptoms, usually precipitated by acute stress (e.g. infection or surgical operation), comprise collapse, shock, hypotension, vomiting and dehydration.

**See if**

- intercurrent illness arises in patients receiving, or just having completed, steroid therapy.

**Action when seen**

| *Assessment* | *Management* |
|---|---|
| Systemic illness, but no vomiting or hypotension | Double dose of oral steroids or, if steroids recently stopped, restart at high dose |
| Systemic illness with vomiting | Hydrocortisone (100 mg) IM every 6 hours |
| Systemic illness with any evidence of dehydration or hypotension | Hydrocortisone (100 mg) IV **Admit** |

**Before leaving**

- remember that patient will need to be reassessed later
- make sure that patient has a steroid card.

# 7.2 Diabetes

## 7.2.1 The New Diabetic

- Generally presents in the surgery because onset tends to be slow enough for patient to be seen routinely.
- Occasional emergency presentation in: pre-existing, undiagnosed diabetic with intercurrent illness; neglected or acute-onset juvenile-type diabetes; socially-isolated old person.
- Presenting symptoms likely to be vomiting, abdominal pain, tachypnoea or symptoms of an intercurrent illness, rather than the classical ones of thirst and polyuria.
- Diagnosis must be considered in any patient where an apparently simple illness is having an unexpectedly severe effect, particularly if there is vomiting, dehydration or ketosis.

**IF THERE IS ANY SUSPICION OF DIABETES, TEST THE URINE OR DO A BLOOD GLUCOSE**

**Action when seen**

| *Diagnosis* | *Management* |
|---|---|
| Made after emergency presentation | **Admit** |
| Made incidentally in mild diabetic | Treat or **refer** in usual manner |

## 7.2.2 The Known Diabetic

The known diabetic will present as an emergency because of intercurrent illness, or hypo- or hyperglycaemia.

### 7.2.2.1 Intercurrent Illness

- All diabetics should be educated to seek medical help for intercurrent illness, especially if there is vomiting or diarrhoea.

**See**

- to treat intercurrent illness and manage its effects on diabetic control

**Telephone advice**

- Before seen
  *The patient must continue with insulin or oral drugs. Make sure that the patient takes plenty of fluids until seen.*

**Action when seen**

- **Assessment**
  - Assess mental state, respiratory rate and hydration.
  - Assess factors relevant to the diagnosis and treatment of the intercurrent illness.
  - Test urine for ketones.
  - Check blood glucose.

- **Management**
  - The same general principles apply whether the patient is on insulin or oral hypoglycaemics.
  - In both cases, changes in dose are necessary if intercurrent illness is producing systemic effects.
  - Do NOT stop insulin or oral drugs: adjust dosage, if necessary.
  - Maintain a large intake of fluid.
  - Maintain carbohydrate intake as far as possible, if necessary by glucose drinks.
  - Treat intercurrent illness appropriately, using antibiotics, where indicated, sooner rather than later.
  - Before every dose of insulin, check blood glucose and adjust dose accordingly.
  - When insulin doses need to be adjusted and frequent blood glucose tests are needed, enlist the help of the local diabetic liaison nurse.

| *Drug* | *Assessment* | *Management* |
|---|---|---|
| Insulin | No vomiting<br>Blood glucose moderately raised | Add 5 units to the soluble component of the normal dose and then adjust according to blood glucose tests |
| | Vomiting but blood glucose not raised | Reduce normal insulin dose by 20%<br>Recheck blood glucose in 4 hours |
| | Marked elevation of blood glucose<br>Persistent ketonuria, signs of dehydration or vomiting not controlled | **Admit** |
| Oral hypoglycaemic | No vomiting but marked glycosuria | Increase drug dose |
| | Difficulty in control | Consider giving a supplement of 10 units of soluble insulin once or twice a day |
| | Persistent ketonuria, signs of dehydration or vomiting not controlled. | **Admit** |

NB: Careful supervision is necessary. The patient must be reassessed before every dose. If this is not possible or you are unwilling to do this, **admit.**

*Remember*

- Patients may refer to marks on the syringe as 'units'.
- When advising changes of insulin dosage, make sure that you and the patient are talking about the same thing.

**Admit if**

- patient is dehydrated
- patient exhibits marked ketosis
- patient is persistently vomiting
- patient is confused
- patient lives in poor social conditions
- you or the patient lack confidence for home management.

**Before leaving**

- ensure that patient will test blood glucose and/or urine for sugar and ketones every 4 hours and inform you of the result if blood levels increase or marked glycosuria or ketones persist
- remember that you must be willing to revisit within 24 hours, otherwise the patient should not be managed at home
- consider using a diabetic clinic liaison nurse (in areas where they exist) to visit the patient at home to check blood glucose and adjust insulin dosages

### 7.2.2.2 Hypo- and hyperglycaemia

- May occur because of neglect of treatment, intercurrent illness, excess insulin, missed meals, unexpected exercise, excess alcohol.
- In practice it is generally hypoglycaemia which presents as an emergency and caller may refer to a 'reaction' or 'funny turn'.
- Remember oral hypoglycaemic drugs can cause hypoglycaemia.
- Hypoglycaemia should be considered as a diagnosis in any patient found confused or semiconscious.
- A known diabetic with any confused, unusual or aggressive behaviour should be considered to be hypoglycaemic until proved otherwise.
- Persistent hypoglycaemia can lead to brain damage so where there is any diagnostic doubt treat as hypo. Treatment will do no harm whereas treatment delay might.

**Visit necessary unless** patient conscious and reasonably cooperative and takes oral glucose or sugar which succeeds in restoring normality.

**Telephone advice**

- Before seeing
  *Try and get the patient to take some sugar before seen.*

**Action when seen**

- **Assessment**

| *Hypoglycaemia* | *Hyperglycaemia* |
|---|---|
| Sudden onset | Slow onset |
| Pale face | Flushed face |
| Sweaty | Dry |
| Full pulse | Weak pulse |
| Aggressive or odd behaviour | Normal behaviour |
| No ketones | Ketones |

- **Management**

| *Assessment* | *Management* |
|---|---|
| Patient conscious and reasonably cooperative | Oral glucose/Hypostop<br>Review treatment and diet |
| Patient unconscious or uncooperative | Glucagon (1 vial) IM, SC or IV<br>When patient recovers (in 5–20 minutes), give oral sugar/hypostop<br>Review treatment and diet |
| Treatment unsuccessful | **Admit** (for IV glucose) |
| Hyperglycaemia (coma or semicoma) | **Admit** |
| If in doubt, treat as hypoglycaemia | |

**Before leaving**

- ensure that patient understands why hypoglycaemia has occurred and what action to take if it recurs.
- prescribe emergency glucagon injection kit and arrange for nearest relative to see practice nurse to be taught how to give injection.

## 7.3 Hypoparathyroidism

- May occur because of accidental removal of, or damage to, parathyroids during a thyroid operation.
- Presents with tetany.
- Symptoms, which are persistent although fluctuating in intensity, are muscle cramps, carpopedal spasm and laryngeal stridor.
- Commonest cause of tetany is hyperventilation (p. 164).

**Admit if**

- acute tetany is suspected to be the result of hypocalcaemia.

## 7.4 Thyroid Diseases

### 7.4.1 Hyperthyroidism

- Occasionally, a thyrotoxic patient may present fairly acutely with palpitations or symptoms of acute anxiety.
- Consider hyperthyroidism as a diagnosis, especially in the anxious patient without relevant psychosocial problems.

**See**

**Action when seen**

| *Assessment* | *Management* |
|---|---|
| Mild or moderate symptoms | Investigate or **refer** routinely |
| Persistent sinus tachycardia (over 120) | Start propranolol (40 mg) TID before investigation or **referral** |
| ANY evidence of cardiac decompensation or recent onset of atrial fibrillation | **Admit** |

### 7.4.2 Myxoedema

- May present as emergency, particularly in neglected or socially-isolated old people.
- Likely reasons for an emergency call are confusion, stupor and coma.
- May also be cause of hypothermia.
- Must be admitted to hospital although the prognosis is very poor.

# 8 ENT Emergencies

*Apart from epistaxis and dental problems, presenting ENT emergencies are more likely to be in children than in adults. In most cases, telephone advice, to tide patients over until they can be seen at the next available surgery, will be more appropriate than a visit.*

## Chapter Contents

## 8.1 Acute Earache

- May be from lesion in ear or pain from a dental problem or neuralgia.
- Careful history should distinguish causes fairly easily.

**See only if**

- pain is severe and persistent
- patient is febrile
- there is any associated vestibulitis or the symptoms of meningitis.

**Telephone advice**

- When no need to see
  *Take suitable analgesics every 4 hours. Do NOT put any drops in the ear. Apply dry heat to the ear and come to the next available surgery. Call again if any new symptoms develop.*

- Before seeing
  *Take painkillers. I will see you later.*

**Action when seen**

| *Diagnosis* | *Features* | *Management* |
|---|---|---|
| Acute otitis media | Follows URTI<br>May be accompanied by hearing loss and/or discharge<br>Often malaise and pyrexia<br>Drum congested and thickened or bulging | Amoxil (250 mg) stat. and TID for 3 days.<br>Simple analgesics every 4 hours |
| Acute mastoiditis | Only occurs after a middle ear infection<br>Pain and pyrexia increase<br>Mastoid area becomes tender, red and oedematous | ANY suspicion, **refer** to ENT immediately |
| Furuncle | Severe pain in outer part of the ear and on moving auricle | Apply dry heat<br>Simple analgesic every 4 hours<br>Consider giving antibiotics |
| Acute otitis externa | Usually past history<br>Smelly discharge<br>Itching<br>Pain<br>Some loss of hearing<br>Tenderness on retraction of pinna | Keep ear canal clean and dry<br>Simple analgesics every 4 hours<br>Topical antibiotic-steroid combination drops or<br>Aluminium acetate 3% wick |
| Traumatic perforation of the eardrum | Generally history of sudden change in air pressure (blow, explosion etc.)<br>Most heal spontaneously | If small and/or non-infected:<br>Seal ear with cotton wool soaked in petroleum jelly<br>Keep ear canal dry<br>Make ENT appointment |

*Continued*

| Diagnosis | Features | Management |
|---|---|---|
| | | If large and/or infected: **Refer** to A & E or ENT urgently |
| Acute barotrauma | Generally has occurred during diving or flying<br>Caused by high negative pressure<br>Pain will decrease in a few hours, when transudate is produced<br>Deafness persists with transudate | If pain severe or persists, **refer** to ENT urgently for incision ear drum |
| Dental causes | Usually obvious if from caries or abscess<br>May be from temporomandibular dysfunction 1–2 months after dental work | Simple analgesics every 4 hours<br><br>If from abscess, Amoxil<br>**Refer** to dentist |
| Glossopharyngeal neuralgia | Short-lived, extremely severe shooting pain extending from ear to throat<br>Pain easily precipitated<br>No abnormalities on examination | Suitable analgesia<br>Consider prescribing Carbamazepine (Tegretol) |
| Malignancy | Malignant disease in the throat may present with referred pain in the ear | In cases of undiagnosed earache, especially in the elderly, **refer** to ENT |

## 8.2 Acute Sinusitis

- History of URTI, dental infection or nasal allergy.
- Characterised by nasal congestion and purulent discharge.
- May be accompanied by fever, malaise and headache.
- If maxillary, teeth may hurt; if ethmoidal, may be swelling near nasal canthus of eye.

**See if**

- pain is severe and persistent
- patient is febrile and/or toxic
- there are any associated symptoms of meningitis.

**Telephone advice**

- When no need to see
  *Take suitable analgesics every 4 hours. If not on MAOI, obtain decongesting nasal spray from chemist and use it with steam inhalations. Make appointment for the next available surgery.*

- **Action when seen**
- **Management** — Amoxil (500 mg) stat. and (250 mg) TID.

## 8.3 Acute Vertigo

- Generally presents with patient complaining of feeling funny, dizzy or lightheaded.
- May be difficult for patient to explain exactly what is being experienced, but vertigo implies a false sensation of rotation or movement.
- In its severest form, may be accompanied by nausea, vomiting, pallor, sweating, disturbed sense of balance and unsteady gait.
- 'Lightheadedness' which is not associated with rotation is non-vestibular in origin, and may be caused by anxiety and/or depression, malaise of fever, syncope, hypoglycaemia or postural hypotension.
- True vertigo is caused by lesions of the labyrinth or its central connections, so, because the cochlea is involved, there may be tinnitus and deafness.

**Visit**

- is justified because symptom is so distressing.

**Telephone advice**

- When about to visit
  *Lie down with your eyes closed and your head still until I arrive.*

**Action when seen**

- **Assessment**
  - Exclude serious disease of the ear or CNS:
    Examine ear carefully and check hearing. NB: If vertigo can be provoked by suddenly increasing the air pressure in the external auditory meatus, invasive middle ear disease is present. This can be done by pushing the tragus firmly and sharply into the opening of the external auditory meatus.
    Check for nystagmus.
    Examine CNS.
    - If no obvious cause check CVS for factors which could predispose to cerebrovascular insufficiency or infarction.

| *Diagnosis* | *Features* | *Management* |
|---|---|---|
| Vestibular neuronitis (epidemic vertigo) | May be caused by viral infection which has produced sudden failure of one labyrinth, with accompanying acute vertigo, nausea and vomiting<br>Movement of head worsens symptoms | Bed rest until dizziness passes<br>Stemetil (12.5 mg) IM and (5 mg) oral TID |

*Continued*

| *Diagnosis* | *Features* | *Management* |
|---|---|---|
| | Horizontal nystagmus usually present, with quick phase to the side opposite lesion<br>Self-limiting condition: worst symptoms will subside within 24–48 hours, although it may be 6 weeks before all symptoms abate | |
| Menière's disease | Mainly affects patients over 50<br>Recurrent attacks of true vertigo, which may last for hours<br>Patient prostrated, with hearing loss and vomiting and/or tinnitus | Bed rest<br>Stemetil (12.5 mg) IM<br>Cinnarizine (15 mg) initially 2 TID |
| Vertigo associated with otitis media or other middle ear disease | Serious symptom, as it suggests fistula formation between inner and middle ear | **Admit** to ENT |
| Vertigo associated with neurological symptoms and signs other than deafness | May be acoustic neuroma, MS or epilepsy<br>If transient likely to be from transient ischaemic attacks | Stemetil (12.5 mg) IM and (5 mg) TID<br>**Refer** to neurologist urgently except if basilar artery insufficiency when should consider prophylactic soluble aspirin |

**Before leaving**

- explain to the patient what is happening and how long the symptoms are likely to persist
- arrange follow-up in 1–2 weeks or sooner.

## 8.4 Foreign Body in the Ear

- Generally occurs in children.
- Damage likely from the foreign body is minor compared with damage likely to result from ill-advised attempts at extraction.

**See**

- **Management**
  - Some foreign bodies (e.g. paper) may be easily removed by syringing, or with blunt forceps or an angled probe (NB: Care must be taken not to drive the foreign body further into the ear.)
  - If foreign body is live insect fill the ear with olive oil or water to drown insect and give relief before removal.

- If patient not likely to be cooperative and sit still or if you are not experienced in using a blunt-angled probe (passed beyond the foreign body and gently withdrawn) and head mirror then **refer** to A & E or to ENT surgeon.

**Before leaving**

- if foreign body has been removed by you, check that the tympanic membrane has not been damaged and that no other foreign body is present in the nose or ears.

## 8.5 Sudden Deafness

- Almost always unilateral.
- May be conductive, from wax suddenly swollen after exposure to water, or from obstruction of eustachian tube.
- May be sensorineural of viral, vascular, traumatic or toxic aetiology, often with obvious history of preceding viral illness or barotrauma.

**See at next surgery**

**Action**

| *Cause* | *Management* |
|---|---|
| Wax | Syringe ear |
| Sensorineural | Urgent ENT **referral,** as patient will probably be **admitted**<br>(Doubtful if any treatment will influence course of events) |

## 8.6 Epistaxis

- Often alarming, rarely dangerous.
- Only the minority of cases—those which have not been successfully treated at home by simple first aid—will be brought to your attention.
- Generally from Little's area (anterior portions of nasal mucosa).
- In the elderly, may be from arteriosclerotic vessels further back in the nose; if so, much harder to control.
- Decide whether to visit on the basis of the age of the patient, patient's general condition, apparent amount of blood lost and what first aid has been tried.
- The majority of cases will be dealt with by advice on appropriate pressure techniques.

**See if**

- the patient is old and possibly arteriosclerotic
- bleeding recurs or persists despite proper use of pressure
- panic engendered will not allow your absence.

**Telephone advice**

- When no need to see
  *Calm down: this is not as bad as it looks. Unless the patient feels faint (in which case, he or she should lie down), he or she should*

*sit up and lean slightly forward. Apply firm, even pressure by pinching the nostrils closed between the thumb and forefinger. Maintain this pressure for at least 5 minutes while the patient breathes through the mouth. Apply a cold compress to the bridge of the nose. When the bleeding stops, the nose must not be blown for 12 hours, and thereafter only gently. If there is no recurrence, no further action is necessary. If bleeding persists or recurs despite pressure, patient must be seen. Generally, best to come to surgery, while pinching the nose, as there are better facilities than at home.*

**Action when seen**

- **Assessment**
  - Release compression and gently clean the nose to see if an anterior bleeding point exists.
  - Check general condition of patient, including pulse and BP.

- **Management**

| *Signs* | *Management* |
|---|---|
| Anterior bleeding point | Diazepam (10 mg) IM, if patient panicky<br>Apply pressure, as above |
| Persistent bleeding despite pressure | If confident, pack nose (see below)<br>If not experienced or posterior bleeding point exists, **refer** to A & E |

## 8.6.1 Packing the Nasal Cavity

- Equipment

  Cotton wool; 4% lignocaine–1:1000 adrenaline; nasal speculum; angled forceps; roll of 0.75-cm ribbon gauze; tube of an oily paste such as bismuth iodoform paraffin paste (BIPP); clean cup; good light.

- Method:

  Soak pledgets of cotton wool in 4% lignocaine–1:1000 adrenaline.
  Insert these into the nasal cavity and wait for 5–10 minutes.
  If bleeding continues when they are removed, firmly pack nose with about 2 metres of ribbon gauze soaked in BIPP.
  Secure a loop of gauze (about 20 cm) to one of the speculum blades.
  Insert speculum, then push loop of gauze about 7–8 cm along floor of nose with angled forceps.
  Build up successive layers of pack from the base to the roof of the nasal cavity.
  Place U-strips of micropore over the nostrils to hold the pack in place.

NB: Do NOT try to pack too far back in the nose, as movement of the soft palate will be liable to dislodge the pack.

- Follow-up:
  After 15 minutes, inspect pharynx.
  If bleeding has not stopped, **admit**.
  If bleeding has stopped, patient must stay propped up in bed and be reviewed in a few hours.
  If there is any recurrence of bleeding, **admit**.
  Otherwise, instruct patient to rest propped up until pack is removed in about 24 hours.

**Before leaving**

- remember that if the bleeds have been severe or recurrent patient must have FBC checked.

## 8.7 Acute Hay Fever

- May present as emergency in young children with sudden onset of swollen face and grossly oedematous eyes.
- Otherwise, you are only likely to be called if hay fever is severe with wheezing.
- Unless this is a fairly clear-cut exacerbation in a patient who has a supply of antihistamines, patient will need to be seen for antihistamines (see treatment of angioneurotic oedema, p. 165) or for treatment for asthma (see p. 159).

## 8.8 Foreign Body in the Nasal Cavity

- Generally occurs in children.
- May be soft and porous, quickly becoming infected and leading to characteristic foul-smelling unilateral discharge.
- May be hard, smooth-surfaced object which does not become infected but may lead to local tissue reaction, with production of much mucus.

**Telephone advice**

*If the patient is an older child and able to cooperate, try to blow the object forcibly down the nostril. If this does not move the object, or if the patient is a young child, come direct to the surgery.*

**Action when seen**

- **Management**
  - If forcible nose-blowing is not effective and the foreign body cannot be easily seen and grasped by forceps or dislodged by angled probe **refer** immediately to ENT surgeon: the foreign body constitutes a definite risk, since it may be inhaled.

## 8.9 Acute Sore Throat

- Generally affects children, but 15–25 year olds may get glandular fever or bouts of streptococcal tonsillitis.

- Cough and runny nose etc. indicate viral infection. Clinically, it is almost impossible to reliably distinguish between streptococcal and viral infections.
- If a bout of acute tonsillitis is followed by severe unilateral pain radiating from the region of the angle of the jaw to the ear, dysphagia and inability even to swallow saliva, this is probably peritonsillar abscess (quinsy).

**See if**

- patient is febrile and/or toxic
- patient is in severe pain so cannot swallow
- there is a possibility of an abscess.

**Telephone advice**

- When no need to see
  *Take plenty of cool drinks. Take available analgesics every 4 hours. If no symptoms of a cold develop, make a surgery appointment.*

- Before seeing
  *Take painkillers until seen.*

**Action on arrival**

| *Assessment* | *Management* |
|---|---|
| Patient febrile and/or toxic with no clear cut signs of a cold | Plenty of fluids and rest<br>Suitable analgesia<br>Start penicillin V course, parenterally if necessarily |
| Suspected abscess (trismus, tonsils grossly enlarged, bulging of soft palate) | Benxylpenicillin (adult dose: 1 megaunit) IM<br>**Refer** to ENT ugently |

## 8.10 Dental Problems

A patient will seek your help because the dentist is unavailable. If you have the telephone number of an emergency dental service, **refer** the patient to it.

### 8.10.1 Toothache

- Attempts to determine the precise cause of dental pain are pointless, except in order to identify factors which may indicate a dental abscess (persistent severe pain localised to affected tooth which is tender to touch, possible facial swelling, pyrexia, malaise).

**Telephone advice**

- When no need to see
  *Take available analgesics in maximum dosage every 4 hours. Apply a pledget of cotton wool soaked in oil of cloves to the offending tooth. Avoid very hot, cold or sweet food or drinks. Contact a dentist at the earliest opportunity.*

**Action when seen**

| *Assessment* | *Management* |
|---|---|
| Possible abscess and dentist unavailable | Prescribe Flagyl and Amoxil but if chemist not available start Amoxil |
| Severe pain | Apply a pledget of cotton wool soaked in 1% lignocaine to the tooth |

## 8.10.2 After an Extraction

- Pain and haemorrhage are the only significant problems.
- Pain may be immediate (due to local trauma) or delayed (due to 'dry socket').
- Bleeding usually mild, but can be serious, so essential to ask about patient's general condition.

**Telephone advice**

- When no need to see

  For pain:

  *Take paracetamol, but not aspirin. Apply local heat or cold to outside of cheek.*

  For bleeding:

  *Position a folded piece of gauze or bandage over the socket and bite on it for 15 minutes. If possible, contact dentist. If you cannot and the bleeding does not stop, call again and I will arrange to see you.*

**Action when seen**

- **Assessment**
  - Check general condition of patient, including pulse and BP.
  - Identify source of haemorrhage.
- **Management**
  - Apply pressure for 15 minutes, as above.
  - If bleeding still not controlled, **refer** to hospital dental department or A & E.

# 9 Eye Emergencies

*Eye disease and trauma form a small, but nonetheless important, part of general practice emergency care. In such a visually-oriented animal as man, the consequences of damage to or loss of sight are so serious that particular care must be exercised in diagnosis and management, thereby avoiding potentially dangerous pitfalls.*

## Chapter Contents

## 9.1 Acutely Painful and/or Red Eye

- Common presenting symptom, usually in the surgery.
- If bilateral, generally conjunctivitis.
- Failure to recognise and treat such conditions as herpetic keratitis or acute glaucoma may result in permanent loss of vision.
- Proper facilities for examination of the eye are vital. Since adequate lighting, binocular loupe, sterile local anaesthetic drops, fluorescein drops or sticks, and ophthalmoscope are all necessary, the patient is best seen at the surgery.

**See urgently unless**

- you are confident that you are dealing with simple conjunctivitis (bilateral; gritty rather than painful; sticky or discharging eyes, whose visual acuity is unchanged).

---

**Telephone advice**

- When no need to see
  *This is very probably conjunctivitis. Keep the eyelids clean with cotton wool and warm water. Do NOT pad the eyes. Come to the next available surgery.*

---

- Before seeing
  *Take an analgesic. Keep the eyes shut, if that is more comfortable, until seen.*

**Action when seen**

- **Assessment**
  - Check for possible loss of visual acuity, past history of eye disease and morning discharge.
  - Carefully examine conjunctiva, pupil and cornea; local anaesthetic drops (amethocaine 1%) instilled prior to examination of painful lesions help greatly.
  - Test visual acuity, if any suggestion that it is impaired.
  - Stain with fluorescein and look at the cornea with a magnifying glass to exclude dendritic ulcer of herpes simplex; ulcers and corneal abrasions will stain green, a green ring will form around a foreign body.
  - Look for any signs of herpes zoster affecting the ophthalmic division of the trigenual nerve.

| | *Acute conjunctivitis* | *Acute iritis* | *Acute glaucoma* | *Keratitis or corneal ulcer* |
|---|---|---|---|---|
| *Pain* | Gritty rather than painful | Moderate, with photophobia | Severe and radiating | Moderate |
| *Discharge* | Often purulent | None | None | May occur |
| *Visual disturbance* | May be smeared with discharge | Blurred | Gross, with haloes round lights | Blurred, if central cornea involved |
| *Site of injection* | Peripheral | Circumcorneal | Diffuse and purplish | Diffuse or circumcorneal |

*Continued*

| | *Acute conjunctivitis* | *Acute iritis* | *Acute glaucoma* | *Keratitis or corneal ulcer* |
|---|---|---|---|---|
| *Pupil and light reflex* | Normal | Small, irregular, poor reflex | Large, oval and fixed | Normal |
| *State of cornea* | Clear | May be hazy | 'Steamy' | May be ulcer (check with fluorescein) |
| *Intraocular pressure* | Normal | Normal | Very high | Normal |

**Management**

| *Diagnosis* | *Management* |
|---|---|
| Acute conjunctivitis | Bathe eye, then instil chloromycetin drops every 1–3 hours<br>Apply ointment to the lower fornix nocte<br>Do NOT pad the eye |
| Acute iritis | **Refer** for urgent ophthalmic opinion<br>If this is not feasible and you are certain of what you are doing:<br>Instil cyclopentolate 0.5% drops every 6–8 hours (for cycloplegia)<br>Corticosteroid drops applied locally<br>Advise oral analgesics before patient is seen by ophthalmologist |
| Acute keratitis | **Refer** for urgent ophthalmic opinion<br>**Never** use steroids before an expert opinion has been obtained |
| Severe (large or central) corneal or dendritic ulceration | **Refer** for urgent ophthalmic opinion<br>**Never** use steroids before an expert opinion has been obtained |
| Corneal abrasion or mild (small or peripheral) ulceration | Instil cyclopentolate 0.5% (1 or 2 drops) and chloromycetin drops or ointment<br>See 24–48 hours to stain eye with fluorescein to check whether corneal epithelium has healed completely |
| Ophthalmic zoster | **Refer** for urgent ophthalmic opinion |
| Acute glaucoma | Temgesic (0.2–0.4 mg) SL<br>**Admit** |

*Never*

- pad a discharging eye
- use local steroid drops before staining the cornea to totally exclude corneal ulceration (particularly the dendritic type)
- use local steroid drops if in doubt about the diagnosis.

## 9.2 Chemical Burns of the Eye

- Alkalis are generally more dangerous than acids.

**Telephone advice**

- When no need to see
  *Wash out the eye with copious amounts of water. If necessary, put the patient's head in a bucket of water, with the eye open. After washing, put a pad over the eye and go to A & E.*

## 9.3 Arc Eye

- Flash burn of the cornea, which causes severe pain, epiploria and blepharospasm.
- Characteristically occurs several hours after exposure to ultraviolet light.
- Most of these burns heal within 24–48 hours.

**Action when seen**

- **Management**
  - Instil amethocaine 1% drops for immediate relief and to allow eye examination.
  - Instil cyclopentolate 0.5% (1 or 2 drops) every 6–8 hours for 24 hours.
    (NB: Accommodation recovers within 24 hours of cyclopentolate).
  - Instil chloromycetin drops every 4 hours.
  - Place pad over eye.
  - Advise paracetamol once local anaesthetic wears off.
  - Re-examine in 48 hours.

## 9.4 Foreign Bodies in the Eye

- Usually dust, sand, metallic grit, wood splinters or tobacco ash.
- History will determine type of foreign body and whether there is ANY possibility of a penetrating injury (e.g. was the patient grinding metal or using a hammer and chisel?)

**Direct for urgent ophthalmic opinion if**

- eye is injured
- there is ANY possibility of a penetrating injury
- foreign body is deeply embedded in the cornea

**Telephone advice**

- When no need to see
  *If washing out the eye with plenty of water does not remove the object, come to the Surgery.*

**Action when seen**

- **Assessment**
  - Give amethocaine 1% drops to relieve pain and to allow examination.
  - Examine eye carefully, including subtarsal area.

- **Management**
  - Attempt to remove the foreign body with moist cotton wool swab.
  - If practised, use hypodermic needle to remove embedded particle.
  - If foreign body successfully removed:
    stain eye with fluorescein to assess damage
    instil chloromycetin drops
    place pad over eye for 24 hours
    see patient in 48 hours to check cornea again.

  If foreign body remains in eye, eye damaged or any possibility of penetration of eye
  **Refer** for urgent ophthalmic opinion

## 9.5 Trauma to the Eye

- May be contusion, abrasion or penetration.
- Contusion may vary from a simple black eye or subconjunctival haemorrhage, to major injury like lens dislocation, rupture of the globe or retinal detachment.
- Abrasion is mainly significant if the cornea is involved.
- Penetration is not always easy to detect. If it is due to a small particle which has entered at high speed (e.g. from metal grinding or chiselling), the patient may have only a vague feeling of 'something in the eye'.

**Refer directly to A & E or see quickly**

**Telephone advice**

- When no need to see
  *If there is ANY suggestion of serious injury, advise going direct to nearest Eye unit.*

- Before seeing
  *If the injury is only minor, cover the eye and come to the surgery for examination.*

**Action when seen**

- **Assessment**
  - Examine surface of eye and under both lids for foreign bodies.
  - Examine and stain cornea for abrasions.
  - Assess visual acuity.
  - Use ophthalmoscope to examine anterior chamber and fundus.

● **Management**

| Assessment | Management |
|---|---|
| ANY major trauma or ANY possibility of a penetrating injury | **Refer** for urgent ophthalmic opinion |
| Minor corneal abrasion | Instil cyclopentolate 0.5% (1 or 2 drops) and chloromycetin drops or ointment<br>See 24–48 hours later to stain eye with fluorescein to check that corneal epithelium has healed completely |

*Remember*
Swollen eyelids or periorbital tissues may conceal serious underlying ocular injuries. Expert advice is needed sooner rather than later.

## 9.6 Sudden Loss of Vision

- May be painful or painless, transient or permanent, unilateral or bilateral.
- May be that the patient has just noticed what has been a gradual loss of vision in one eye.

**See urgently**

**Telephone advice**
- Before seeing
  *Try to keep calm. I will see you soon.*

**Action when seen**

● **Assessment**
- Examine visual acuity.
- Assess visual field.
- Perform full examination of the eye.

| Diagnosis | Features | Management |
|---|---|---|
| Temporal arteritis (see p.131) | Consider in all middle-aged and elderly patients<br>May be history of headaches, loss of weight, malaise, aches and pains | **Admit** for confirmation of diagnosis and high dose steroids |
| Optic neuritis | Consider in younger patient with ocular discomfort and tenderness with pain on eye movement<br>Only sign may be loss of central visual acuity, although disc atrophy may follow<br>Pupil on affected side may react poorly to light | **Refer** for urgent neurological opinion<br>Generally, no treatment necessary, and good recovery of vision is expected |

*Continued*

| *Diagnosis* | *Features* | *Management* |
|---|---|---|
| Central retinal artery occlusion | Complete, painless loss of vision<br>Pupil on affected side dilates and does not react to light<br>Fundus pale and oedematous, with 'cherry red spot' on fovea | **Refer** urgently |
| Central retinal vein occlusion | Pathognomonic fundal picture of extensive intraretinal and pre-retinal haemorrhage and distention of retinal veins | No treatment available<br>Patient to attend next ophthalmic outpatients |
| Vitreous haemorrhage | If severe, may cause sudden loss of vision in one eye<br>If non-traumatic, likely to be secondary to retinal tear or pre-retinal neovascularisation (from any condition associated with widespread ischaemia, e.g. diabetes) | **Admit** |
| Retinal detachment | May be preceded by flashing lights or multiple floaters<br>May be history of trauma or high myopia<br>Visual field defect or, if macula involved, sudden, severe, central loss | **Admit** |
| Migraine | May be preceded by unusual and alarming visual field defects, followed by severe headache and nausea<br>Diagnosis obvious, unless this is the first attack | p. 130 |
| Maculopathies | Painless loss of central vision<br>May be subtle macular changes, hence precise diagnosis difficult | Obtain urgent ophthalmic opinion, unless you can diagnose with confidence, in which case routine ophthalmic **referral** |
| Cortical blindness | Sudden loss in one or both eyes may be due to damage to posterior visual pathway<br>Generally vascular in nature<br>Usually emergency treatment is of no avail | **Refer** for urgent neurological evaluation |
| Hysteria | Relatively common<br>Usually tunnel vision which cannot be accounted for on clinical grounds | Consider if psychiatric **referral** is indicated |

## Notes

# 10 Forensic Emergencies

*The police and police surgeons deal with the vast bulk of emergencies where there may be forensic problems. They are the experts and we shall not attempt to cover situations that properly come under their jurisdiction. Rape, murder and grievous bodily harm are not matters to be dealt with by GPs, although occasionally GPs do become involved peripherally or, more especially, with 'shocked' relatives. Death at home is the main area where an alert GP's suspicions may be aroused and where, even for routine certification, the GP has to know the correct legal procedure. Accordingly, death at home is the only area we cover in detail.*

## Chapter Contents

## 10.1 Alleged Assault

- In most cases, the victims of assault will be first attended to in A & E or by the police.
- When the GP is involved, it is often because of the emotional reaction of those close to the victim, rather than because of the victim's clinical state.
- This reaction may well be out of proportion to the actual injuries received and more concerned with obtaining a medical witness than with obtaining treatment.

**See if**

- injuries received require treatment that may be appropriately given by you.
- emotional uproar is such that your absence will not be tolerated, and your presence will be calming.

**Telephone advice**

- When no need to see
  Advise if A & E and/or police should be involved rather than you.
  If a record is required rather than treatment, arrange to see the victim at a place and time convenient to you.

- Before seeing
  *Try to keep calm until seen.*

**Action when seen**

- **Assessment**
  - Attempt to gain full and clear history.
  - Perform a full physical examination.
  - Make detailed notes of all injuries.
- **Management**
  - Treat injuries appropriately.
  - ANY puncture wounds or stab wounds must be seen by a surgeon.

**Before leaving**

- Consider, in the light of the injuries that you have just treated, if and when it would be appropriate to see the patient again.

## 10.2 Alleged Indecent Assault

- Call is generally from the distraught parent of a child who may have been indecently assaulted.
- Call comes when the parent learns of the incident; this may be some time after it occurred.
- Try to persuade callers to involve the police immediately as if examination necessary should be carried out by trained person.
- Consider whether in the public interest you ought to contact the police.

**See only if**

- family refuse to involve police
- your presence is necessary to manage emotional reactions—usually in relatives rather than the victim

- **Action when seen**
- **Assessment**
  - Take history calmly and sympathetically.
  - Allow the child to talk without continual parental interruption.
  - Perform careful external physical examination

---

- **Management**
  - Encourage parents to contain emotional reactions in front of the child as this may easily aggravate any emotional trauma suffered.
  - If history/examination suggests an assault has actually taken place then repeat advice to involve police and/or consider whether you should involve social services.
  - Make clear and comprehensive notes.

---

**Before leaving**

- advise the parents not to keep bringing the subject up with the child and not to treat the child differently, especially if the incident appears to have been minor or capable of being interpreted in more normal ways
- offer a routine appointment in a few days time for a further chat.

## 10.3 Alleged Rape

- Police and police surgeon should be involved from the outset.
- Unless forensically trained, examination by you is likely to confuse rather than help the resolution of the problem.
- Relatives and friends may need support and help and be allowed to ventilate their feelings.
- Once the initial police investigation is over, the victim will need support, sympathy and understanding for a considerable period of time.
- Make sure STDs have been excluded.
- Prescribe postcoital contraception, if appropriate. If too late for this exclude pregnancy.

## 10.4 Death at Home

- Whether dramatic and unexpected, or a long-awaited event in a chronically ill patient, death will still have a considerable emotional impact on the relatives.
- Although the caller may think that the patient is dead, you can only tell by visiting and examining the body. Until you have given your official diagnosis, all concerned are in limbo.
- Apart from diagnosing death, you can give helpful practical advice to the living to guide their actions.

**Visit quickly unless**

- it is an expected institutional death
- it is an expected death in the middle of the night, and those in attendance are happy for examination of the body to wait until morning.

**Telephone advice**

- When about to visit
  *I shall be with you as soon as possible.*

**Action when seen**

- **Assessment**
  - Is the patient dead?
    Death is indicated by
    - absent pulse
    - absent heart sounds (in the case of drowning or electrocution, you may have to listen for up to 5 minutes to ensure that there is no life)
    - fixed and dilated pupils
    - absent corneal reflexes
    - engorged retinal vessels.
  - Are the circumstances of death in any way suspicious?
    Is the body obviously injured?
    Is the body lying in a strange way or unusual situation?
    Is there poison or another means of suicide apparent?
  - Can a death certificate be issued?
    Doctor examining the body must be satisfied that death was by natural causes.
    Patient's doctor must have been in professional attendance during the last 14 days of the last illness (this does not apply to Scotland) and must think that he or she knows what the (natural) cause of death was.
  - Need the Coroner/Procurator Fiscal be informed?

**Circumstances under which the Coroner/Procurator Fiscal must be informed**

| *Do NOT issue death certificate if* | *Issue a death certificate if you wish (mark BOX A on reverse) if* |
|---|---|
| ● doctor did not attend during the last 14 days of the patient's life<br>● cause of death unknown or uncertain<br>● violent death<br>● death to which an accident contributed<br>● death to which anaesthetic or operation contributed<br>● doubtful stillbirth | ● death from industrial disease<br>● death in a patient with a pensioned disability<br>● death from poisoning or drugs (including alcohol)<br>● death by suicide<br>● death as a result of illegal abortion<br>● any criticism of patient's medical or nursing care appears likely<br>● death from want, exposure or neglect |

*Remember*

Do NOT omit vital information from a certificate for any reason. It is a legal document deserving due care and attention.

- **Management**

| *Assessment* | *Management* |
|---|---|
| ANY suspicion of foul play or suicide | Move nothing<br>Do NOT interfere with the body or the scene<br>Call the police |

*Continued*

| *Assessment* | *Management* |
|---|---|
| Natural causes | Tell the relatives that the patient is dead<br>Give suitable sympathy and commiserations<br>Advise if and when a death certificate can be issued<br>If a death certificate cannot be issued, tell relatives about the involvement of the Coroner/Procurator Fiscal and inform him or her or the police |

- If the Coroner/Procurator Fiscal becomes involved, he or she will take over the issuing of the death certificate.
- Give simple, easily followed advice to relatives about contacting an undertaker and any other questions they may wish to have answered.
- Do not be embarrassed about allowing your emotions to show if you were emotionally involved with the patient.

**Before leaving**

- ensure that the relatives understand when and where a death certificate can be collected
- ensure that the relatives appreciate that you are available should they wish to contact you to talk about what has happened and how they are going to feel about it.

## Notes

# 11 Gastrointestinal Emergencies

*Acute abdominal pain is the most important emergency presenting symptom in the gastrointestinal system. In general practice, it is the only presenting symptom that is more likely to have a serious than a trivial cause. It is also unusual in that the formation of a precise diagnosis is not as important as making the correct management decision as to whether the condition requires surgery, and hence urgent admission.*

## Chapter Contents




See also Hiccups, p. 168
See also Testicular pain, p. 175

# 11.1 Abdominal Pain

## 11.1.1 General Approach

- Acute abdominal pain always causes anxiety in patients and relatives because of the fear that it may signify the presence of some surgical condition, such as appendicitis.
- You may also feel this anxiety, as your first duty is to exclude such a condition.
- Beware of bias: even the most chronically neurotic, anxious and depressed patients can suffer from surgically correctable pathology.
- Beware of the apparent gastroenteritis that turns out to be appendicitis.
- Obtain information about the time of onset, nature and severity of the pain, so that you can assess the degree of urgency.

**See unless**

- pain is clearly colicky associated with diarrhoea.
- absolutely clear from story that symptoms are minimal. Even then best to get caller to report back in 1–2 hours so situation can be reassessed.

**Telephone advice**

- Before seeing
  *The patient must not eat or drink anything before seen.*

**Action when seen**

- **Assessment**
  - Careful history will often reveal the diagnosis before any examination.
  - Is the patient toxic or obviously in severe pain?
  - Take temperature and pulse.
  - Perform careful and leisurely abdominal examination.
  - Listen to bowel sounds, feel hernial orifices and perform rectal examination.
  - Examine other systems, if you think that this may be helpful.
  - Is this a surgical condition requiring urgent admission?

| *Acute surgical condition* | *Medical or cold surgical condition* |
|---|---|
| Pain of recent onset | Recurrent pain |
| Constant pain | Colicky pain |
| Marked tenderness | Little or no tenderness |
| Rebound tenderness | No rebound tenderness |
| Fever | Apyrexial |
| Toxic or shocked | Not toxic or shocked |

NB: Definite guarding implies surgical condition

● **Management**

| *Assessment* | *Management* |
|---|---|
| Acute surgical condition | **Admit**, even if you cannot make a precise diagnosis |
| Medical or cold surgical condition | Keep patient under observation until the pain subsides<br>Try to reach a precise diagnosis |

## 11.1.2 Making a Diagnosis

*Remember*

- The GP sees cases early in their development, when symptoms may well be atypical. In many cases, reassessment and reconsideration will be necessary before you can reach a diagnosis.
- Your main objective is to identify those cases needing immediate hospital treatment, rather than to make a clever diagnosis.

- Is the pain generalised and colicky?

| *Diagnosis* | *Features* |
|---|---|
| Acute or sub-acute obstruction (adhesions, carcinoma, strangulated hernia, volvulus etc.) | Severe and increasing colic<br>Vomiting, constipation and abdominal distension<br>Increased, then absent or tinkling bowel sounds<br>PR reveals empty rectum |
| Gastroenteritis | Vomiting and diarrhoea worse than pain |

- Is the pain generalised, severe and persistent?

| *Diagnosis* | *Features* |
|---|---|
| Peritonitis | Patient toxic<br>Severe and widespread tenderness and guarding |
| Perforated peptic ulcer | Severe pain of sudden onset in upper abdomen<br>Shocked patient with rigid abdomen |

- Is the pain localised and colicky?

| *Diagnosis* | *Features* |
|---|---|
| Acute gastritis | Epidemic or induced by alcohol<br>Epigastric tenderness and pain |
| Gall-stones | Severe pain in right hypochondrium, which may radiate into back, chest and epigastrium |
| Renal colic (stones or infection) | Pain in loin, radiating into iliac fossae or perineum<br>May be haematuria, dysuria etc. |
| Dysmenorrhoea | Suprapubic pain, possibly radiating into lower back or legs |

- Is the pain localised and persistent?

| *Site of pain* | *Diagnosis* | *Features* |
|---|---|---|
| Upper abdomen | Peptic ulcer | Recurrent pain<br>May be hunger pains, relieved by antacids<br>Moderate tenderness only |
| | Hepatitis | Nausea<br>Jaundice<br>Tender liver |
| | Cholecystitis | May be history of gall-stone colic<br>Fever<br>Tender gall-bladder |
| Central or iliac fossae | Pancreatitis | Central boring pain may extend to back<br>Often seen in alcoholics<br>May be marked tenderness and guarding |
| | Aneurysm | Central pain or backache<br>Pulsatile mass |
| | Crohn's disease | Tender mass in RIF may present as sub-acute obstruction |
| | Appendicitis | Always number one suspicion<br>Central pain, moving to RIF<br>Local tenderness, guarding and rebound<br>OFTEN ATYPICAL |
| | Diverticulitis | Recurrent pain<br>Occurs in the old<br>Tender descending colon |
| | Ischaemic bowel | Occurs in the older arteriosclerotic patient<br>Vomiting and/or diarrhoea<br>Marked tenderness |

*Continued*

| *Site of pain* | *Diagnosis* | *Features* |
|---|---|---|
| | Ulcerative colitis | Occurs in young patients<br>Diarrhoea with blood<br>Patient may be acutely toxic |
| Lower abdomen | Pelvic abscess | Results from appendix or gynaecological infection<br>Fever<br>Tender mass PR or PV |
| | Pelvic inflammatory disease | Pain possibly with fever and purulent discharge.<br>Tenderness of uterus or tubes on PV |
| | UTI | Dysuria, frequency<br>Suprapubic tenderness |
| | Miscarriage | History of pregnancy symptoms or amenorrhoea<br>Vaginal bleeding before pain |
| | Ectopic pregnancy | Patient may not even have missed period<br>Pain before vaginal bleeding<br>Patient may be shocked |
| | Ovarian cysts | If torsion, acute pain and tenderness<br>Otherwise, mass abdominally or on PV |

## 11.1.3 Management of Specific Disorders

| *Diagnosis* | *Management* |
|---|---|
| Biliary colic | Temgesic (0.4 mg) SL<br>Treat at home, unless conditions poor<br>If pain persists for more than a few hours, **admit** |
| Acute cholecystitis | Temgesic (0.4 mg) SL **and** (if much vomiting) Maxolon (10 mg) IM<br>If pain relief good, treat at home and start broad-spectrum antibiotic<br>If patient toxic or pain persists, **admit** |
| Acute pancreatitis | Cyclimorph (15 mg) IM<br>**Admit** |
| Perforated ulcer | Cyclimorph (15 mg) IM or IV<br>**Admit** |
| Peritonitis | Cyclimorph (15 mg) IM<br>**Admit** |
| Acute appendicitis<br>Acute or sub-acute obstruction<br>**ANY** undiagnosed pain with tenderness and guarding | Even if you only suspect the diagnosis, **admit**<br>If patient shocked or in severe pain, or a long journey to hospital is likely, consider giving IM analgesia |

Renal colic, see p. 174.
Gynaecological conditions, see p. 143.

**Before leaving**

- remember that if the patient is staying at home you must be prepared to revisit and reassess
- advise patient if further investigation e.g. cholecystogram or surgical outpatient opinion will be necessary.

## 11.2 Food Poisoning or Gastroenteritis

- Presents as vomiting and diarrhoea of acute onset.
- Whatever the aetiology, the management is the same.
- Most patients accept episodes of vomiting and diarrhoea as part of life, and cope without seeking medical advice.
- Emergency call may be for advice or visit, usually because patient feels awful or fears 'food poisoning'.
- Ascertain patient's occupation, as this will influence the length of time before a return to work is allowed, e.g. food handlers should not return to work until stool cultures are negative.

**See if**

- patient is elderly
- patient lives alone
- patient does not readily accept your telephone advice
- patient appears to be ill
- pain predominates or is persistent rather than colicky and intermittent

---

**Telephone advice**

- When no need to see
  *These symptoms generally clear in about 48 hours.*
  *Increase intake of clear fluids, little and often, even if vomiting persists. Avoid eating solids until the vomiting ceases. If vomiting persists for more than 24 hours or if new symptoms develop, call again.*

---

- Before seeing
  *Take only clear fluids until seen.*

**Action when seen**

- **Assessment**
  - Assess general state of patient, particularly hydration
  - examine abdomen to exclude appendicitis.

---

- **Management**
  - Advise patient as for telephone advice.
  - Maxolon (10 mg) IM if vomiting is severe and persistent or its effects are socially unacceptable e.g. in an elderly isolated or immobile patient.

---

## 11.3 Haematemesis

- The sight of blood in vomit is alarming.
- Majority of cases are due to peptic ulceration.

- History of alcohol and/or analgesic ingestion may be relevant.
- Violent vomiting may rupture a small blood vessel in the oesophagus or throat so that fresh blood appears in the vomitus.
- Obtain some idea of the amount of blood loss and the general state of the patient.

**See unless**

- it is clear that only a few streaks of blood have been mixed with the vomit.

**Telephone advice**

- Before seeing
  *Keep what has been vomited so I can see it.*

**Action when seen**

- **Assessment**
  - Attempt to assess amount of blood vomited.
  - Check pulse, BP, colour of patient as pointers to extent of internal bleeding.
  - Ascertain if there is any melaena.
- **Management**

  Unless bleeding has clearly been caused by the action of vomiting, **admit** (medical)

**Before leaving**

- ensure that you will be called if there is any recurrence of bleeding or if patient feels ill or faint or if stools become black.

## 11.4 Jaundice

- Rare presenting symptom, since it is much more likely to be noticed by the doctor then the patient.
- Occasionally, patient may notice change in colour of skin, urine or stools, and seek urgent advice.
- New cases in the young are especially due to viral hepatitis.
- In the middle-aged or older patient, consider drug reactions, gall-stones or malignancy as possible causes.

**See if**

- it is a newly presenting case

**Telephone advice**

- Before seeing
  *Collect a urine sample for me to test.*

**Action when seen**

- **Assessment**
  - Take full medical and social (including alcohol and job) history.
  - Ascertain if any drugs have been taken recently.
  - Perform full physical examination, especially of skin, abdomen (liver, ascites) and PR.
  - Look for injection sites if drug addiction suspected.
  - Note urine colour; testing is of little value if blood tests are going to be performed.
  - Take, or make arrangements for blood samples, for ESR, FBC and LFTs.

| *Diagnosis* | *Signs* |
|---|---|
| Hepatocellular disease (e.g. infective hepatitis, alcohol, drugs) | Gradual onset over 1–2 weeks, with anorexia and malaise, followed by mild jaundice and production of dark urine and pale stools. In the young, assume infective hepatitis |
| Obstructive jaundice (e.g. gall-stones, malignancy) | Gradual, painless onset of deep jaundice, with very pale stools and pruritus. Sudden onset with pain and/or fever suggests gall-stones, with cholecystitis or pancreatitis. |

- In many cases, diagnosis is not as clear cut as appears from the table. Rarely, cases of haemolytic jaundice present suddenly.

**Management**

- The main decision is whether to **admit**. If there is no pain, fever or obvious liver failure, there is no harm in waiting for a day or two before reviewing the biochemistry and seeing how the jaundice is developing.

| *Assessment* | *Management* |
|---|---|
| Hepatocellular disease | Bed rest<br>No alcohol<br>Light carbohydrate diet<br>No drugs, other than simple antiemetics<br>ANY complications, consider specialist **referral** |
| Obstructive jaundice, with pain or fever | **Admit** |
| Obstructive jaundice, without pain or fever | Surgical **referral** |

**Before leaving**

- remember that the patient staying at home will need clinical and biochemical follow-up
- if infectious hepatitis is diagnosed fill in a notification of infectious disease form.

## 11.5 Perineal Pain

- Patients are often not very good at localising pain in the perineum; a paid 'down below' may refer to anywhere from coccyx to pubis.
- May be from anal abscess, Bartolin's cyst, piles, anal fissure or testicular problems, so attempt to locate the pain exactly.

**Visit if**

- pain is obviously severe
- patient is distressed or immobile.

**Telephone advice**

- When no need to see
  *Take aspirin or paracetamol. Attend the next surgery.*

- When seeing
  *Take aspirin or paracetamol. I will see you later.*

**Action when seen**

- **Assessment**
  - Most perineal pains are due to conditions which are visible.
  - Perform PR and PV as indicated.
- **Management**

| *Diagnosis* | *Features* | *Management* |
|---|---|---|
| Bartholin's abscess | On posterior aspect of vaginal introitus, on either side | **Admit** for incision and/or marsupialisation |
| Pilonidal sinus | Occurs in males<br>Recurrent in midline posteriorly | Broad-spectrum antibiotic |
| Perianal abscess | Red, tender swelling lateral to rectum | Surgical intervention, as appropriate |
| Perianal Haematoma | Blood blister on anal margin | Analgesics and rest<br>If pain is severe, incise |
| Prolapsed pile | Very tender lumb protruding from rectum | Push back into rectum<br>If this cannot be done, advise local anaesthetic ointment and rest |
| Anal fissure | Spasm of sphincter<br>Fissure visible | Local anaesthetic ointment<br>Dilatation later if needed |
| Proctalgia fugax | Recurrent<br>Worse at night<br>No signs | Digitally stretch puborectalis muscle<br>Analgesia<br>Colofac TID<br>High fibre diet |

*Continued*

| *Diagnosis* | *Features* | *Management* |
|---|---|---|
| Bladder calculus | Dysuria<br>Haematuria | See p. 174 |
| Prostatitis | Urinary tract symptoms<br>Possible urethral discharge<br>Tender PR | Analgesia<br>Broad-spectrum antibiotic |
| Pain in testicle | Epidymo-orchitis<br>Torsion | See p. 175 |

## 11.6 Rectal Bleeding

- Patients seem to be remarkably tolerant about rectal bleeding, ascribing it to 'piles': take the call seriously.
- Ascertain if it is fresh blood or melaena, how much has been lost, and if there is any diarrhoea or abdominal pain.

**See if**

- there is moderate bleeding
- there appears to be melaena
- patient has any associated symptoms, such as abdominal pain, fainting.

**Telephone advice**

- When no need to see
  *Make a routine appointment. If the bleeding recurs or becomes heavier, call again.*

- When about to visit
  *Lie the patient down until I arrive.*

**Action when seen**

- **Assessment**
  - Assess amount of blood lost and patient's general condition.
  - See if there is a visible bleeding point.
  - Perform PR to discover if melaena or carcinoma are present.

- **Management**

| *Signs* | *Management* |
|---|---|
| Visible bleeding point | Dress with firm pad<br>Apply pressure with bandage or sanitary towel |
| Malaena | **Admit** |
| Substantial bleed (any cause) | **Admit** |
| Fresh blood with abdominal pain | Likely to require **admission** |
| Small amount of fresh blood | Instruct patient to stay at home and contact you if the bleeding persists, in which case **admission** is likely to be required |

**Before leaving**
- ensure that the patient appreciates that surgery follow-up is necessary.

## 11.7 Umbilical Bleeding or Discharge

- Common request for telephone advice because patient may think that bleeding from the umbilicus is connected with the bowel.

**Telephone advice**
- When visit not necessary
  *Do not worry. This does not indicate any internal trouble. Clean the navel regularly with surgical spirit and a cotton bud.*

## 11.8 Vomiting

- Distressing symptom for which patients will ask for help not so much because they are worried, but because they feel so awful.
- Significance depends on any associated illness.
- Ask how long this has been happening, how frequently and what is being vomited e.g. coffee grounds
- Ask specifically about vertigo, severe headache, confusion, abdominal pain, constipation and diarrhoea.

**See unless**
- it is clear from the history that the vomiting is being caused by uncomplicated gastritis or gastroenteritis.

**Telephone advice**
- When no need to see
  *Increase the patient's intake of clear fluids, taken little and often, even if the vomiting persists. Do not take any solids until the vomiting settles. If vomiting persists for more than a few hours or if new symptoms develop, call again.*
- Before seeing
  *Take sips of clear fluid only until seen.*

**Action when seen**

- **Assessment**
  - Assess general state of patient, including hydration.
  - Take history and examine to exclude as possible causes ENT infection, raised intracranial pressure or meningism, bowel obstruction or acute abdomen, migraine, anxiety, hepatic or renal failure, drugs or infections.

**Management**
- Treat any underlying condition.
- Do not use antiemetics for vomiting *per se* unless you are reasonably certain of what is going on. If used inappropriately, they may mask or obscure developing pathology.
- Advise extra clear fluids and observe.

## 11.9 Diarrhoea

- Not usually the sole symptom precipitating the call, but, if so, probably because the presence of blood or persistence (especially in children).
- If uncomplicated, most unlikely to need to be seen, but make sure that you understand exactly what the patient means by diarrhoea.
- Assess frequency, duration and associated symptoms.

**See if**

- patient is obviously toxic
- this is a persistent symptom in the elderly or chronic sick.
- pain predominates or is persistent rather than colicky and intermittent.

**Telephone advice**

- When no need to see
  *Increase the intake of clear fluids and if you wish take no food for the next 24 hours. If diarrhoea persists, make routine appointment. If new symptoms develop, call again.*

## 11.10 Worms

- Discovery of a worm in a bowel motion or on the bottom may precipitate a panic call for advice.
- Usually threadworms, rarely roundworms.

**Telephone advice**

- When no need to see
  Threadworm
  *Do not worry. These are not in any way harmful or dangerous. Buy Pripsen or Vermox from the chemist and treat your whole family.*

  Roundworm
  *Do not worry. These are not likely to be harmful or dangerous. It may be an earthworm which has crawled up into the lavatory pan through a crack in the sewer pipe. Make a surgery appointment and bring the worm with you.*

# 12 Musculoskeletal Emergencies

*The detailed management of fractures, dislocations and other acute traumatic conditions is beyond the scope of this book. The large majority of emergency cases involving trauma find their way to hospital either directly or by ambulance, and the GP is unlikely to be involved in any way. Some GPs specialise in the management of accidents involving severe trauma, and a rural GP may be the only person available to help. However, it is fair to say that most GPs would arrive at an accident only by chance and would confine themselves to simple first aid while awaiting the arrival of the more experienced ambulance crew.*

## Chapter Contents



See also Pulled elbow syndrome, p. 46.

## 12.1 First Aid at an Accident

**Management**

- Ensure that the airway is clear.
- If comatose, place the patient in the recovery position.
- Control any bleeding by firm bandaging over a pad.
- Cover any wound with a clean dressing.
- Provide some sort of immobilisation for a fractured limb.
- Keep the patient comfortable until the ambulance arrives.

- Temporary immobilisation of the long bones of the lower limbs is best achieved by bandaging the legs together: in the case of the upper limbs, it is best to bandage the injured arm to the chest.
- When moving a patient with a fractured limb, pain will be lessened by applying traction to the limb while it is being moved.
- If there is ANY suspicion of a fracture of the spinal column, flexion and extension of the spine MUST be avoided. For transport, the patient should be lifted bodily onto a firm surface.
- The analgesic of choice is Cyclimorph IV, although this is absolutely contraindicated if the patient has been unconscious or if there is any history to suggest severe abdominal injury. If an analgesic is given, write the dose and time administered on a note which should be pinned to the patient's chest or handed personally to one of the ambulance crew.

## 12.2 Head Injury

- Majority of cases for which you will be contacted will involve children or the elderly; adults tend to go directly to A & E.
- Call for help may be at the time of injury or later, if symptoms subsequently develop.
- Presenting symptom may have nothing to do with the head injury, but may have been wrongly assumed to be a result of it.
- Accurate history is vital, in order to obtain details of the accident and to determine whether the patient was unconscious at any time and whether the patient is confused, unconscious or vomiting.
- May be difficult to obtain history in children, as often there are no adult witnesses to the accident.

**Direct to A & E if**

- patient was unconscious at any time
- circumstances of the accident indicate the possibility of serious injury
- there is persistent vomiting, headache, confusion or amnesia.

**Otherwise visit**

- especially the elderly or disabled, or examine at surgery soon.

**Telephone advice**

- When no need to see
  *Go direct to A & E: an X-ray may be necessary and the patient may need to be kept in hospital for observation.*

- Before seeing
  *Rest until seen.*

**Action when seen**

- **Assessment**
  - Take history again, in particular to confirm that the patient was not unconscious.
  - Check level of consciousness, pupil reflexes.
  - Examine skull; ears and nose for CSF and/or blood.
  - Look for aetiological factors, especially in elderly patient with head injury from fall, as these may be treatable (e.g. hypotension from drugs, arrhythmias, Stokes–Adams attacks).
  - In children, consider the possibility that child abuse has occurred.
- **Management**

| *Assessment* | *Management* |
|---|---|
| ANY suspicion that the patient was unconscious | **Refer** to A & E |
| ANY abnormal findings in the CNS which are thought to be due to the head injury | **Refer** to A & E |
| Normal history and examination | Advise those in attendance:<br>*If the patient goes to sleep in next 4 hours, rouse him hourly to ensure that he is not unconscious.*<br>*If the patient starts vomiting, becomes confused or develops severe headache, any disorder of speech, vision or co-ordination, take him directly to A & E.* |

**Before leaving**

- make a careful note of your findings and instructions for medico-legal reasons.

# 12.3 Fractures

## 12.3.1 General

- If a patient is unable to stand or walk after an injury, or is unable to use the injured part, this must always arouse the suspicion of a fracture.
- History of visible bruising appearing a day or so after an accident is also suggestive of fracture.
- In many cases, history alone does not provide reliable evidence on which to distinguish between a fracture and a simple strain.

*Remember*

- In fatigue or pathological fractures, there may be sudden onset of pain and disability without any causative injury.

- The patient with a fracture may retain the use of a painful limb, especially with impacted fractures (neck of humerus, neck of femur, lower end of radius), fractures of carpal bones (scaphoid), fatigue and greenstick fractures.

**Direct to A & E if**

- fracture appears likely from the history
- possibility of a fracture demands an X-ray.

**Otherwise visit**

- especially the elderly or disabled, or examine at surgery.

**Telephone advice**

- When no need to see
  *Go direct to A & E; an X-ray will probably be necessary, as may bandaging or plastering. There is little point in me seeing the patient first.*

- Before seeing.
  *Keep the patient comfortable until seen.*

**Action when seen**

- **Assessment**
  - Look for objective signs of fracture: visible or palpable deformity, local swelling, visible bruising, marked local bone tenderness, marked impairment of function.
  - Abnormal mobility or crepitus are diagnostic.

- **Management**

| *Assessment* | *Management* |
|---|---|
| ANY suspicion of fracture | **Refer** to A & E |
| No fracture | Advise:<br>suitable rest<br>analgesia<br>bandaging |

## 12.3.2 Fracture of the Neck of the Femur

- The commonest fracture that you are likely to be called out to see.
- Occurs most often in elderly women.
- May occur spontaneously or after a trivial injury.
- May not present until several days after the event, either because the patient took to bed to wait for the pain to recede, or because fracture is impacted and the patient has been able to walk.
- Consider this diagnosis in any elderly patient who suddenly has difficulties walking.

**Visit**

**Telephone advice**

- Before seeing
  *Do not try to walk on the sore leg. Rest in a comfortable position in bed until I arrive.*

**Action when seen**

- **Assessment**
  - If acute, assess general condition of the patient.

- Look for shortening of the leg and limitation of external rotation.
- Limitation of external and internal rotation may be the only physical sign, especially when impacted.

● **Management**

| *Assessment* | *Management* |
|---|---|
| ANY suspicion whatsoever of fracture | **Refer** to A & E for X-ray and possible **admission** |

## 12.4 The Locked Knee

- Sudden onset associated with strain.
- Due to torn cartilage, although in older patients may be due to a loose body in the joint.
- Knee locks at about 30° of flexion, with tenderness over the associated collateral ligament.

**Visit**

● **Management**

- Manipulation:
  steady the femur with the left hand
  hold the ankle with the right hand and exert lateral or medial pressure to 'open' the affected side of the joint
  maintaining this pressure, rotate the tibia backwards and forwards on the femur, while extending the knee.
- If successful
  rest knee in extension, with supportive bandage teach quads exercise and arrange follow-up.
- If unsuccessful
  **refer** to A & E.

## 12.5 Acute Back Pain

- Fairly common cause of emergency call, as pain may be severe and alarming, leading patient to seek urgent help.
- May arise from mechanical disorders or systemic disease of the spine.
- Rarely, may be referred pain from systemic disease (e.g. peptic ulcer, myocardial infarction).
- Determine severity and distribution of the pain, and if there is any past history.
- Patient's degree of mobility is a good indication of the seriousness of the condition.

**See urgently if**

- pain is severe or root pain exists
- symptoms of other disease are present
- caller does not readily accept advice.

**Visit if**

- patient is immobilised/cannot get to surgery.

**Telephone advice**

- When no need to see
  *Rest on a firm bed and take suitable dose of analgesics every 4 hours. A hot bath or a hot water bottle applied to the back may help. Make an appointment or call again if the pain does not diminish.*

- Before seeing
  *Let the patient rest in whatever position is most comfortable until seen.*

**Action when seen**

- **Assessment**
  - Look for neurological signs.
  - Confirm diagnosis.

| *Diagnosis* | *Features* |
|---|---|
| Mechanical disorders (e.g. prolapsed disc, muscle spasm, ligament tears) | Often a history of trauma<br>Pain relieved by rest, but aggravated by movement, standing or coughing<br>Spine movements usually asymmetrically restricted<br>Tender muscles or ligaments<br>May be evidence of root pressure e.g. sensory loss, loss of reflexes, difficult micturition |
| Systemic disease affecting the spine (e.g. crush fracture, malignancy, infection) | Pain not relieved, or even worsened, by rest<br>Spine movements usually symmetrically restricted<br>May be other evidence of systemic disease |
| Referred pain (e.g. from gynaecological cause, peptic ulcer, prostate) | Spine movements fairly free and movement does not affect pain<br>May be muscle spasm<br>Evidence of other disease |

- **Management**

| *Assessment* | *Management* |
|---|---|
| Moderate backache | Try to keep as mobile as possible.<br>Dihydrocodeine (30 mg) oral stat.<br>Prescribe analgesic and diazepam if necessary (for muscle spasm) |

*Continued*

| *Assessment* | *Management* |
|---|---|
| Severe backache | Rest in position of maximum comfort (for up to 2 days)<br>Temgesic (0.4 mg) SL<br>Prescribe analgesics and diazepam if necessary (for muscle spasm) |
| Backache with nerve root pressure | As above, depending on severity of pain<br>Careful follow-up assessment and investigations necessary |

In some patients, additional treatment might include:

- Injection:
  Lignocaine (5 ml) mixed with Deltastab (1 ml) injected into any localised area of acute tenderness in the back muscles.
- Manipulation:
  May be helpful following acute-onset pain in a young patient with no evidence of root pressure or systemic disease.
  If you do not know how to manipulate, suggest that the patient sees an osteopath.

**Admit if**

- there is bilateral nerve root pressure
- there is any difficulty with micturition
- there is severe pain which is not alleviated by analgesics
- there is severely restricted mobility in a patient living alone
- there is evidence that the cause may be malignancy or systemic disease affecting the spine

**Before leaving**

- give the patient some idea of how long the backache may be expected to last, and how long normal activities are likely to be restricted.
- arrange for follow-up.

## 12.6 Acute Neck Pain

- Differential diagnosis and management generally the same as for acute back pain (see p. 115)
- Meningism can present as acute neck pain

**See if**

- pain is severe or root pain exists
- patient is immobilised
- caller does not readily accept advice
- any suspicion of subarachnoid haemorrhage.

**Telephone advice**

- When no need to see
  *Rest and take a suitable dose of analgesics every 4 hours. A hot bath or a hot water bottle applied to the neck may help. Make an appointment or call again if the pain does not diminish.*

- Before seeing
  *Let the patient rest in whatever position is most comfortable until seen.*

**Action when seen**

| *Dysfunction* | *Features* | *Management* |
|---|---|---|
| Muscle spasm from viral myalgia or pain secondary to infected cervical glands | Slow onset<br>Very tender muscle | Rest neck in collar[1]<br>Advise suitable analgesia<br>If adenitis, treat appropriately |
| Joint dysfunction | Sudden onset<br>Severe pain on movement | Apply traction to neck[2]<br>Rest neck in collar[1]<br>Advise suitable analgesia |

[1] The cervical collar helps to rest the acutely painful neck. In an emergency, one can be made by rolling a newspaper to make a flat band, wide enough to immobilise the neck when placed round it like a parson's collar. Hold the collar in place with a scarf or bandage.

[2] Traction may give quick relief to someone with a 'stuck' neck. Seat the patient on a low stool or coffee table. Standing behind them, put one hand under the chin and the other under the occiput. Steadily pull upwards, keeping the neck straight. If the pain is worsened, STOP. If the pain is relieved, repeat several times before putting on the collar.

## 12.7 Acute Pain Around the Shoulder Joint

- Pain limiting all movements both active and passive indicates acute arthritis or capsulitis.
- Pain arising from the muscles, tendons or bursa round the shoulder joint if limiting mainly active movements the problem limited to muscles or tendons involved.

**See if**

- pain obviously severe.

**Telephone advice**

- When no need to see
  *Use available analgesics every 4 hours. Try the effects of local heat (hot water bottle). Make an appointment for the next surgery.*

- Before seeing
  *Use available analgesics. I will see you later.*

**Action when seen**

- **Assessment**
  - Exclude acute arthritis of the joint, which causes severe restriction of movement in all directions.

- **Management**
  - Prescribe a non-steroidal anti-inflammatory drug plus analgesic as necessary.
  - Advise rest followed by mobilising passive movement.

- If painful arc indicates bursitis or supraspinatus tendonitis then mix Deltastab (2 ml) with lignocaine 1% (4 ml) and inject into the subdeltoid space. (Instruct the patient to sit with the arm hanging down and internally rotated. Introduce the needle between the humerous and the acromium. It should pass medially and upwards at an angle of about 20° to the horizontal.)

## 12.8 Pain Radiating Down the Arm or the Leg

- May be the presenting symptom, but the possible underlying cause should determine your action.

| *Cause* | *Features* |
|---|---|
| Referred pain from spine | Mostly affects the proximal half of the limb<br>Pain distribution does not match nerve root area |
| Referred pain from viscera | No associated musculoskeletal or neurological signs |
| Pain due to nerve root irritation | Severe intractable pain, following nerve root distribution<br>Associated neurological signs |
| Ischaemic pain | Pain worse peripherally<br>Associated with cold limb and absent pulses<br>Elevation of the limb makes it pale and the pain worse |

## 12.9 The Acutely Painful Joint

- Commonest aetiological factor is trauma, although this may just be a provocative factor in a joint with some pre-existing underlying disease (e.g. gout osteoarthritis).
- May be history of gout or systemic disease that might predispose to acute joint pain (e.g. haemophilia).
- May be severe pain in a single joint of a patient with pre-existing polyarthritis.

**Direct to A & E if**

- trauma was severe and patient is badly hurt.

**Otherwise see**

**Action when seen**

| *Diagnosis* | *Features* | *Management* |
|---|---|---|
| Acute ligament tears | Tender periarticular ligaments<br>Immediately painful | Support the joint and rest<br>If severe, **refer** to A & E for X-ray |
| Haemarthrosis | Rapid swelling of joint after trauma | **Refer** to A & E |
| Traumatic synovitis | Gradual onset effusion after trauma<br>May be underlying joint disease | Support the joint and rest<br>Prescribe non-steroidal anti-inflammatory drug |
| Gout or pseudogout | May be past history<br>Hot red joint, usually at the base of the big toe | Dihydrocodeine (30 mg) oral or Diclofenac (75 mg) IM<br>Prescribe indomethacin<br>Arrange follow-up |
| Septic arthritis | Red, very hot, intensely painful joint<br>Fever<br>Rapidly progressive | Temgesic (0.4 mg) SL<br>**Admit** |

## 12.10 Acute Polyarthritis

- Occasionally presents as an emergency.

**See unless**

- these are pains associated with a known viral illness or with an allergic (urticarial) type of rash.

**Telephone advice**

- When no need to see
  *Rest in bed until the pain subsides. Take aspirin or paracetamol. Make an appointment for the next surgery, although if you feel unable to come out request a routine visit.*

- Before seeing
  *Rest until seen.*

**Action on arrival**

| *Diagnosis* | *Features* | *Management* |
|---|---|---|
| Reiter's syndrome | Usually occurs in young males<br>May be history of STD contact or acute diarrhoea<br>Mainly affects knees and ankles | **Refer** to rheumatologist |
| Viral infection | Rubella<br>Infectious hepatitis | Maintain high fluid intake<br>Take analgesics, as necessary |

*Continued*

| *Diagnosis* | *Features* | *Management* |
|---|---|---|
| Allergic reaction | Commonest cause of acutely painful joints | Take analgesics, as necessary<br>Antihistamines orally or IM |
| Rheumatoid arthritis<br>Collagen disease | Affecting smaller joints<br>May be fever | **Refer** to rheumatologist urgently |
| | Acute onset, with systemic illness | **Admit** |
| | Single joint exacerbation | Consider injection of Deltastab (1 ml) into joint<br>Prescription for anti-inflammatory drug |
| Polymyalgia rheumatica | Not true polyarthritis<br>Widespread pain and stiffness, especially of upper limb girdle<br>Great malaise<br>Muscles very tender | Take blood samples for ESR and FBC<br>Prednisolone (20 mg) oral stat. and repeat in 12 hours<br>See again in 24 hours, and reconsider diagnosis if patient not much better |

**Notes**

# 13 Neurological Emergencies

*Symptoms arising from malfunctions of the central nervous system are often dramatic and tend to be very frightening both for patients and those in attendance. Acute changes in consciousness, motor power or sensation usually signify serious disease and should be taken seriously by the doctor as well as by the patient.*

*In an emergency, it is often difficult to arrive at an accurate diagnosis and one has to be concerned with immediate management. Details of differential diagnosis are therefore only given as far as is necessary for deciding the best immediate course of action.*

*The caller must be advised how to put an unconscious patient into the recovery position, thus greatly reducing the risk of asphyxia before your arrival. To save repetition in the text, we use the phrase 'Turn the patient on one side' as shorthand for the instructions regarding the recovery position. The full advice implied is:*

---

*Ensure the airway is clear, remove any dentures or vomit from the mouth.*
*Turn the patient onto his/her side.*
*Draw up the uppermost leg until the thigh is at right angles to the body.*
*Draw up the uppermost arm until it is at right angles to the body with the elbow bent.*
*If the breathing is noisy, put you hand under the chin and gently lift it so that the neck stretches back.*

---

## Chapter Contents



See also Head injury, p. 112

## 13.1 Stroke

- Cerebral haemorrhage, thrombosis or embolus which results in damage to the CNS which persists for 24 hours or more.
- Main aetiological factors are arteriosclerosis, hypertension and emboli from endocardial infarction or mitral valve disease.
- Of patients who suffer from a stroke, 50% die within one month, 25% are left with severe disability and 25% are left with minor disability.
- Often the caller has made the diagnosis and says 'I think that he has had a stroke'.

**Visit**

**Telephone advice**

- When about to visit
  *Keep the patient quiet and lying down until I arrive.*

**Action when seen**

- **Assessment**
  - Assess level of consciousness and damage to CNS.
  - Look for predisposing factors (e.g. hypertension).

- **Management**

| *State of patient* | *Management* | |
|---|---|---|
| Unconscious | **Admit unless** | • death is imminent |
| Severely disabled | **Admit if** | • patient is confused<br>• there is inadequate nursing care at home<br>• those in attendance wish it<br>• underlying cause needs treatment e.g. atrial fibullation, high BP<br>• dedicated stroke unit available. |
| | **Home Care if** | • patient is relatively alert<br>• there are good home facilities<br>• those in attendance are willing to cope<br>• patient wishes to stay at home<br>• no underlying cause needing treatment |
| | Advise rest for 24 hours<br>Arrange nursing help to start mobilisation next day<br>Arrange rehabilitation at day hospital, physiotherapy etc.<br>Treat BP, if necessary | |
| Mildly disabled | **Home care unless**<br>Treatment—As above | • poor social conditions |
| Evolving stroke | **Admit if** | • the stroke is mild initially and slowly becomes worse (this implies oedema, haemorrhage or neoplasm) |

**Before leaving**

- remember that the patient who stays at home will need a revisit next day, or sooner if condition deteriorates.
- Evaluate risk factor for reocurrence and make management plans for secondary prevention.

## 13.2 Transient Ischaemic Attack

- Caused by microemboli or sudden decrease in blood flow in arteriosclerotic vessels.
- Produces dysfunction in the part of the brain served by that particular vessel.
- If in carotid territory, there may be hemiparesis, dysphasia, loss of vision in one eye and sensory loss.
- If in vertebro-basilar territory, there may be motor defects, dysarthria, ataxia, vertigo, drop attacks and transient loss of consciousness.
- By definition, attacks are transient, and patient will recover fully within 24 hours.
- Important symptom because it heralds established stroke in the future in a substantial number of cases.

*Remember*

- Transient neurological symptoms (usually visual), followed by a throbbing headache, may be a migraine attack. This is easy to diagnose in a younger patient with history of migraine. However, if this is the first-ever migraine attack, it is difficult to distinguish from TIA or even subarachnoid haemorrhage.

**See**

**Telephone advice**

- Before seeing
  *Needs to be seen quickly. Lie the patient down until seen.*

**Action when seen**

- **Assessment**
  - Carefully assess CNS.
  - Measure BP and examine fundi.
  - Examine CVS, looking for arrythmias, carotid bruits or valvular heart disease that could cause emboli.
  - Check urine for sugar.
- **Management**

| *Assessment* | *Management* |
|---|---|
| No obvious treatable cause | Rest for 24 hours<br>Aspirin (150 mg) oral daily<br>Follow up—if recurrent—refer |
| Identified probable cause of embolism | Give aspirin<br>Refer/admit urgently |
| Severe hypertension | **Admit** |
| Obvious cause for transient hypotension (e.g. arrhythmia) | Treat/refer appropriately |

**Before leaving**

- reassure the patient that this is not a proper stroke and that recovery is likely to be complete.
- arrange for follow-up and further investigation as necessary.

## 13.3 The Persistently Unconscious Patient

- Sinister symptom necessitating a quick response.
- Patient often elderly, so caller will be very alarmed.
- May be the result of head injury, stroke, meningitis, diabetes, hypothermia, poisoning or the terminal stage of any illness.
- In practice, accurate diagnosis is often not possible, so your role will be to give immediate first aid and arrange for **admission.**

**Visit unless**

- It is more appropriate to send for an ambulance urgently and it is likely to get there before you.
- this is an expected event in a terminal illness, and you do not feel that a visit, to give support, is necessary.

**Telephone advice**

- When about to visit
  *Turn the patient on one side. I shall be with you as soon as possible.*

**Action when seen**

- **Assessment**
  - Ensure that the patient's airway is clear.
  - Perform general examination, looking for signs of head injury, low body temperature, stroke, neck stiffness.
  - Look for evidence of diabetes (e.g. drugs, injection marks, diabetic card, medic alert bracelet).
  - Look for evidence of drugs or alcohol overdose.
- **Management**

| *Assessment* | *Management* |
|---|---|
| ANY possibility of hypoglycaemia | Glucagon (1 vial) IM<br>If patient recovers, give sugar/ Hypostop orally<br>If not, **admit** |
| Expected terminal event | Comfort relatives<br>Arrange for nursing help, if needed<br>Offer to call again in a few hours or sooner, if the patient dies |
| All other cases | **Admit** |

## 13.4 Transient Loss of Consciousness

- 'Blackouts' are alarming and often give rise to emergency calls.
- Even a simple faint may cause panic: surprisingly few people know how to handle the situation.
- For practical purposes, the differential diagnosis is between a fit and a faint, though in the elderly, transient ischaemic attacks may cause a transient loss of consciousness (see p. 125).
  *Remember*
  Hypoglycaemia may produce rapid, transient loss of consciousness.

| *Fit* | *Faint* |
|---|---|
| Usually occurs with no warning | Patient feels dizzy or faint before losing consciousness |
| May be specific aura | No aura |
| Patient does not go pale | Patient goes pale |
| Strong pulse | Weak pulse during attack |
| Patient often incontinent | Patient rarely incontinent |
| Convulsive movements | Convulsion only occurs if the faint is prolonged (e.g. by keeping patient upright) |
| Patient sleepy or confused after fit | Patient rapidly returns to normal, if allowed to lie down |

### 13.4.1 Faint (Syncope)

- Usually the result of a vasovagal attack associated with erect posture, warmth, nervous tension or some sudden unpleasant sensation.
- Commonest in young females near time of period.
- May be due to fall in BP due to arrhythmias, aortic valve disease, myocardial infarction or drugs.
- Micturition syncope may occur in elderly patient who gets out of bed, usually in early hours of the morning, to pass water.
- Cough syncope may occur with severe bout of coughing.
- Hyperventilation syncope may occur with hysterical overbreathing (see p. 164).
- Calm caller to find out if patient has fully regained consciousness. If so, obtain details about the circumstances of the attack and relevant history.

**See if**

- patient has not recovered properly
- there were any convulsive movements
- there is any history of chest pain, palpitations or breathlessness
- elderly patient who does not usually faint
- clear history is unobtainable.

**Telephone advice**

- When no need to see
  *Keep patient lying down for about half an hour. Call again if the patient faints again, or if any other symptoms develop. The patient can see me at the next available surgery, if so desired.*

- Before seeing
  *Lie the patient down. If unconscious, lie the patient on one side, remove false teeth and loosen collar. I shall be with you shortly.*

**Action when seen**

- **Assessment**
  - If patient still unconscious or semiconscious, ensure that the airway is clear, then put the patient into the recovery position.
  - Carefully assess CNS and CVS, including standing and sitting BP.
  - Ask if the patient is on any drugs.

- **Management**

| *Assessment* | *Management* |
|---|---|
| Young patient<br>Isolated attack<br>Obvious predisposing factors<br>Normal examination | Reassure and explain<br>No further action necessary |
| Older patient<br>Recurrent attacks<br>May be disease of CVS | Keep patient lying down for a while<br>Arrange follow-up and investigation |
| ANY evidence of acute myocardial ischaemia or persistent arrhythmia<br>(NB: Possible silent infarct) | Treat appropriately<br>See section on CVS (p. 54) |

## 13.4.2 Fit

- Beware of the hysterical fit with dramatic jerking movements, often accompanied by shouting and hitting out at people, but no true clonic movements.
- Tetanic carpopedal spasm may be mistaken for a fit, but there are no clonic movements.
- Important to find out if the patient is a known epileptic and to what extent recovery from the fit has taken place.
- In some epileptics increased frequency of fits may be due to drug toxicity, especially to phenytoin, and advice to give an extra dose of medication may be harmful.

**Visit unless**

- patient is a known epileptic and has recovered from the fit.

**Telephone advice**

- When no need to see
  *Make routine surgery appointment for review of therapy, but call me if there are any more symptoms.*

- Before seeing
  *If patient is still fitting, protect him or her from injury. If patient is unconscious, lie him or her on side and clear any vomit from the mouth. I shall be with you shortly.*

**Action when seen**

| *Assessment* | *Management* |
|---|---|
| Patient still fitting | Diazepam (10 mg) IV slowly<br>**Admit** |
| Suspected hysteria | Stroke eyelashes unexpectedly or press firmly over supraorbital nerve. Any reaction from patient indicates that he or she is not unconscious.<br>Firmly tell patient and audience that this is not a fit. Do not be surprised if they do not believe you.<br>If necessary, apply a very wet cold flannel to patient's face |
| Patient unconscious, or if there are any abnormal neurological signs | **Admit** |
| Patient has recovered with no abnormal neurological signs | If this was a first fit it is very important to try to obtain as clear a description as possible from an eyewitness. |

**Before leaving**

- if the patient has recovered, arrange surgery follow-up and ensure that you will be called again if any more symptoms develop.

## 13.5 Headache

- Frequent diagnostic problem in the surgery, but fairly unusual emergency presentation, hence more worrying in this context.
- Difficult to assess on the telephone and you will need full details about previous attacks and any current illness.
- Even if the patient is well known to you and has regular headaches which do not substantially differ from this one, you should ask yourself: why have they called this time?

**See unless**

- patient is a well-known sufferer from headaches not substantially different from this one.

**Telephone advice**

- When no need to see
  *Take usual analgesics. Lie in a darkened room. If headache worsens or other symptoms develop, call me again.*

- Before seeing
  *Lie in darkened room until seen.*

**Action when seen**

| *Cause* | *Characteristics* | *Management* |
|---|---|---|
| Tension headache | Very common<br>Unusual to present as an emergency<br>Bilateral frontal or occipital<br>No other physical signs, apart from tension<br>Often a manipulative procedure | Give firm advice about the nature of the pain, and the appropriate place and time for consultation |
| Migraine | Usually a history of previous attacks or positive family history<br>May have typical transient neurological symptoms before headache<br>Often vomiting<br>No physical signs | Stemetil (25 mg) PR, later dihydrocodeine (30 mg) oral<br>If very severe:<br>Temgesic (0.2–0.4 mg) SL or Imigran IM<br>Stemetil (12.5 mg) IM<br>If possible avoid giving an injection as this sets a precedent for future attacks |
| Cluster headaches | Form of migraine<br>Attacks come in clusters<br>Severe pain with stuffy nose or watering eye | If possible avoid giving an injection as this sets a precedent for future attacks<br>Consider prophylactics Pizotifen (sanomigram) |
| Fever | Any fever, particularly some virus infections, may give quite severe headache<br>Exclude meningitis | Simple analgesics |
| Sinusitis | Usually with URTI<br>Nasal discharge<br>Fever<br>Very tender over the sinus | Simple analgesics and inhalations<br>Prescribe antibiotic |
| Meningitis | Fever<br>Bursting headache<br>Vomiting<br>Meningism | Benzylpenicillin (1.2 g in 8 ml water IV or 4 ml water IM) IV or IM<br>**or** if penicillin allergic chloramphenicol (1 g in 2 ml water) IV or IM<br>**Admit** |
| Encephalitis | Encephalitis often associated with virus infections like mumps | **Admit** |

*Continued*

| *Cause* | *Characteristics* | *Management* |
|---|---|---|
| Sub-arachnoid haemorrhage | Sudden onset<br>Patient often confused<br>May become semiconscious or comatose<br>Meningism | **Admit** |
| Malignant hypertension | Rare<br>May present as headache associated with loss of vision or other symptoms due to cerebral vasospasm.<br>Very high BP<br>May be papilloedema and proteinuria | **Admit** |
| Temporal arteritis | Severe unilateral pain<br>Very tender temporal artery<br>Often history of recent muscular pains | Prednisolone (30 mg) oral<br>Prescription for oral prednisolone<br>Arrange follow-up, ESR etc. |
| Space occupying lesion | Slowly progressive<br>Does not usually present as an emergency unless vascular accident in the tumour<br>May present as vomiting | **Admit** |
| Occipital headache | Pain in the occipital area<br>Associated with cervical spondylosis or with a recent whip-lash injury<br>Often anxiety about the injury | Simple analgesics. Encourage active and passive mobilisation |
| Glaucoma | The severe retro-orbital pain may present as a 'headache'<br>Loss of some vision<br>Hazy cornea | **Admit** |

## 13.6 Oculogyric Crises

- Attacks of neck retraction with upward deviation of eyes.
- Majority of cases are due to toxic reaction to drugs (e.g. phenothiazines, Maxolon).
- In a susceptible patient, crisis may occur after taking only 1 or 2 tablets.

**See**

**Action when seen**

- **Management**
  - Atropine (0.3 mg) SC
  - Diazepam (10 mg) oral
  - Withdraw the drug that is responsible

## 13.7 Pain in the Face

- Severe pain in the face is a not uncommon cause of a call for advice or visit.
- Most such pains do not have a serious cause and the aim of advice or seeing the patient is to relieve pain and distress.
- Dental abscesses can be very painful, and it is useful if you can direct the patient to the nearest out-of-hours dental service (if one exists in your area).

**See if**

- patient is in severe pain or obviously distressed
- cause is dental abscess and no dentist is available
- there is a possibility of ophthalmic zoster.

**Telephone advice**

- When no need to see
  *Take aspirin or paracetamol every 4 hours. Make an appointment to be seen at the next available surgery.*

- Before seeing
  *Take aspirin or paracetamol. I shall see you later.*

**Action when seen**

| *Cause* | *Features* | *Management* |
|---|---|---|
| Dental abscess | Severe throbbing pain<br>Swelling of the jaw<br>Pain on percussing the affected tooth | If dentist unavailable:<br>Dihydrocodeine (30 mg) oral<br>Prescribe Amoxil and Flagyl |
| Sinusitis | Maxillary (pain in the face) | Simple analgesia<br>Inhalations<br>Prescribe antibiotic |
| Herpes zoster | Burning pain, which may be quite severe **before** the rash appears<br>If the ophthalmic division of the fifth nerve is involved, may affect the eye | Dihydrocodeine (30 mg) oral<br>Prescribe analgesics<br>Watch for rash to appear<br>If eye is involved, **refer** urgently or **admit** |
| Trigeminal neuralgia | Sudden, transient shooting pains affecting one division of the fifth cranial nerve<br>Pain provoked by stimuli such as chewing or cold | Prescribe analgesics and Tegretol |
| Glossopharyngeal neuralgia | Pain similar to above, but near angle of jaw and usually not so severe | Prescribe analgesics and Tegretol<br>Exclude ear and cervical gland disease |
| Bell's palsy | Moderate pain over all of one side of the face may herald an attack of Bell's palsy | See next section (Weakness of the face) |

## 13.8 Weakness of the Face

- Usually the cause of much anxiety, because the patient suspects a stroke.

**See urgently**

**Action when seen**

- **Assessment**
  - Examine the face.
  - Perform full CNS examination, if indicated.

| *Upper motor neurone lesion* | *Lower motor neurone lesion* |
|---|---|
| Incomplete paralysis | Often severe paralysis |
| Patient can wrinkle brow and close eye | Patient cannot wrinkle brow or close eye |
| Brisk reflexes | No reflexes |
| Possible causes: stroke, focal CNS lesion, brain tumour | Possible causes: Bell's palsy, herpes zoster of geniculate ganglion, middle ear infection |

- **Management**

| *Assessment* | *Management* |
|---|---|
| Stroke | See p. 164 |
| Suspected focal CNS lesion or brain tumour | Urgent neurological **referral** |
| Bell's palsy | Prednisolone (20 mg) stat. and prescribe high-dose descending course<br>Reassure that this is not a stroke<br>Arrange for follow-up in a few days |
| Herpes zoster | Acyclovir (800 mgs) 5 times daily<br>Arrange for follow-up in a few days |
| Middle ear infection | Urgent ENT **referral** or admission |

## 13.9 Sudden Weakness of the Legs

- May be from spinal cord compression (disc prolapse, tumour), spinal cord thrombosis or polyneuritis.
- Often symptomatic of a funtional illness, but patient must be examined to exclude a physical cause.

**Visit**

**Action on arrival**

- **Assessment**
  - Perform careful CNS examination to determine if a physical cause is present.
- **Management**
  - ANY evidence of spinal cord damage **admit**

**Notes**

# 14 Obstetric and Gynaecological Emergencies

*Vaginal bleeding and abdominal pain are undoubtedly the two most significant presenting symptoms in this system. Differential diagnosis, assessment and management differ, depending on whether the woman is pregnant, and, if so, how far on.*

*Nearly all GPs provide full antenatal and postnatal care for their patients, but very few provide intrapartum home care other than in an emergency. Unfortunately, all GPs, whether on the Obstetrics list or not, have an unequivocal obligation to provide maternity medical services in an emergency. Unless faced with something straightforward, with which you are used to dealing, we suggest that you advise the patient to seek specialist help and that you offer to make the necessary arrangements.*

*In some districts, effective obstetric flying squads exist, making it feasible, in certain clinical situations, to resuscitate the patient before subjecting her to the trauma of an ambulance journey. In other districts, where there may be no flying squad or only a nominal, ineffective service, it will be safer and quicker to summon an ordinary ambulance. You must be aware of the standard of the emergency obstetric services in your area, and act accordingly.*

*Unless an extreme situation exists, where whatever your experience you have to do your best, you should never attempt any procedure where lack of expertise, suitable equipment or suitable working conditions might lay you open to legal or professional criticism. If a patient insists on staying at home, it may be necessary to ask a consultant obstetrician to carry out an urgent domiciliary consultation.*

## Chapter Contents

# 14.1 Pregnancy and Childbirth

## 14.1.1 General Factors

- Good antenatal care helps to decrease the likelihood of emergency calls.
- Always ask for date of LMP to ensure that patient is pregnant and, if so, to estimate period of gestation.
- Remember: many disorders present atypically during pregnancy.
- Because she is pregnant, do not assume that the patient's symptoms are being caused by her condition.
- Abdominal pain requires the same general approach as in the non-pregnant.
- Bleeding PV is frightening, as there are natural fears of damage to or loss of the foetus.
- Make an estimate of the amount of blood lost from the number of sanitary towels used (internal or external), passage of clots and general condition of the patient.
- In general, you should have good reasons for not seeing the patient, rather than the other way round.

## 14.1.2 First Trimester

- Most common time for emergency calls, as about 15% of pregnancies end in early abortion.
- If periods irregular or only overdue by 1–2 weeks, history of nausea, vomiting, frequency, sore or tingling breasts, and constipation may help clinical diagnosis.
- If a parous patient thinks that she is pregnant again, she is probably right.
- Pain occurs after bleeding in abortion and hydatidiform mole, but it is the first symptom of ectopic pregnancy.
- Always have at the front of your mind ectopic pregnancy as a possible diagnosis, particularly in pregnancy arising from failure of IUCD or the progestogen-only pill.

**See**

- unless this is mild bleeding in early pregnancy which is not associated with pain.

**Action when seen**

- **Vaginal bleeding**

| *Diagnosis* | *Features* | *Management* |
|---|---|---|
| Threatened abortion | Painless, mild bleeding<br>Gentle VE confirms that cervical canal is closed | Bed rest until bleeding stops<br>Ask to be recalled if pain starts or blood clots are passed |
| Incomplete, inevitable abortion | Threatened, followed by intermittent pain in lower abdomen and back | **Admit**<br>If bleeding is severe, remove products from vagina or |

*Continued*

| *Diagnosis* | *Features* | *Management* |
|---|---|---|
| | Cervix dilates and products of conception are extruded into cervical canal and vagina<br>Gentle VE confirms cervical dilation | cervical canal, and give Syntometrine (1 ml) IM before ambulance arrives |
| Complete, inevitable abortion | As above, but bleeding and pain will have stopped because all products of conception have been expelled | Either **admit** for D & C or, if you are sure that all products have been expelled, observe at home and **admit** if bleeding starts again<br>If not admitted check blood group and give anti-D if Rh. neg. and gestation more than 12 weeks |
| Septic abortion | Signs of infection (fever, smelly discharge)<br>ANY suspicion of illegal interference | **Admit** |
| Hydatidiform mole | May present as abortion Often patient is big for dates and may have excess vomiting or signs of PET<br>May pass vesicles PV | **Admit** |

NB: Bleeding may also be caused by a local lesion (e.g. polyp, carcinoma of the cervix, cevicitis, varicosities). If seen at home, a speculum examination is not usually practical. If painless bleeding persists, and it is not severe enough to warrent admission, the patient should be seen in the surgery for a speculum examination to exclude local causes. Management of painless bleeding from local causes is the same as for threatened abortion.

- **Abdominal pain**

| *Diagnosis* | *Signs* | *Management* |
|---|---|---|
| Ectopic pregnancy | 1 in 300 pregnancies are ectopic<br>Cramp-like pain in either iliac fossa in patient with early symptoms of pregnancy<br>May be associated with fainting and/or passage of some dark blood | If classical story, do NOT VE<br>**Admit** |

*Continued*

| *Diagnosis* | *Signs* | *Management* |
|---|---|---|
| | The pain usually precedes the bleeding<br>NB: May not be definite history of amenorrhoea, especially if IUCD *in situ* or on progestogen-only pill | |
| Torsion ovarian cyst | May occur as uterus rises out of pelvis (rupture of lutein cyst may also occur in the same manner)<br>Acute pain with local tenderness | If suspected, **admit** |
| Acute pelvic infection | Usually associated with gonococcal infection or criminal interference | **Admit** |

## 14.1.3 Second Trimester

- Vaginal bleeding and abdominal pain are the main presenting symptoms.

**Action when seen**

- **Vaginal bleeding**
  - Assessment as for the first trimester, although the cause is unlikely to be ectopic pregnancy.
  - If bleeding is trivial and no pain see in surgery to examine perineum and vagina for local cause of bleed.
  - If bleeding is significant, **admit**.
- **Abdominal pain**

| *Diagnosis* | *Signs* | *Management* |
|---|---|---|
| Acute UTI | Often silent, but may present with classical features of pyelonephritis | If pyelonephritis, **admit**<br>If cystitis with no systemic upset, manage at home, take MSU specimen, maintain high fluid intake<br>Prescribe Amoxil |
| Red degeneration of fibroid | Acute pain<br>Tenderness<br>Swinging temperature | **Admit** |

*Remember*

During the second trimester, appendicitis may be particularly difficult to diagnose because of atypical presentation.

### 14.1.4 Third Trimester

- Bleeding at this stage is antepartum haemorrhage and not abortion, so NEVER perform VE at home.
- Fulminating PET or eclampsia with fit may rarely present in patient with concealed pregnancy or who has not been receiving antenatal care.

**Action when seen**

- **Vaginal bleeding**

| *Diagnosis* | *Features* | *Management* |
|---|---|---|
| Placenta praevia | Recurrent painless bleeding from placenta, encroaching on lower segment<br>May be associated malpresentation | Do not perform VE<br>**Admit** |

- **Abdominal pain**

| *Diagnosis* | *Features* | *Management* |
|---|---|---|
| Accidental haemorrhage (abruption) | Continuous severe abdominal pain<br>Haemorrhage mainly retroplacental and concealed, but usually some vaginal bleeding<br>Tender and hard uterus<br>Patient's condition poor and out of proportion to the amount of blood apparently lost<br>Foetus may be dead | If clear history, call ambulance before visiting<br>Cyclimorph (10–15 mg) IV<br>IV infusion, if available<br>**Admit** |
| Premature labour | Pain in lower back, radiating round to the front<br>May be show or rupture of membranes | **Admit** |

- **Other presenting problems**

| *Diagnosis* | *Features* | *Management* |
|---|---|---|
| Premature rupture of membranes | Gush of liquor with or without signs of onset of labour | VE to ensure cord not prolapsed<br>**Admit** |
| Pre-eclampsia and eclampsia | Unrecognised hypertension, oedema, proteinuria followed by generalised | If PET, **Admit**<br>If patient is fitting ensure that the airway is clear and place |

*Continued*

| *Diagnosis* | *Features* | *Management* |
|---|---|---|
| | headache, visual disturbances and epigastric discomfort | patient in the recovery position<br>Diazepam (10 mg) IV slowly |
| | This may be followed by a fit | **Admit** with oxygen<br>Travel with patient unless obstetric flying squad have taken over management. |

## 14.1.5 Emergency Childbirth

- Occasionally occurs after concealed pregnancy.
- Call may be for abdominal pain or even after the child has been born.
- If presents as emergency childbirth, ensure that an ambulance is sent for before you leave for the patient.
- If the patient is in the second or third stage of labour, you must make the best of a bad job and complete the delivery.
- Obviously, all sorts of complications can occur, and if initial assessment reveals breech delivery, twins or prolapsed cord etc., call obstetric flying squad immediately.

**Action when seen**

- **Management**
- **Normal, second-stage labour**

- Lie patient on her back with her feet supported on the bed.
- Perform VE to see if there is full dilation of the cervix. If there is not, do NOT allow pushing. Confirm vertex presentation and position; ensure that the cord has not prolapsed; assess the pelvic size in relation to the size of the foetal head.
- Place your hand on the perineum to resist too rapid an advance of the head until the head remains widely distending the vulva and no longer recedes between contractions.
- Keep the head flexed until the occiput is well free of the anterior part of the vulva and the nape of the neck is hitched beneath the symphysis. Complete the delivery of the head between contractions. As soon as the head is born, feel along the baby's neck to see if the cord is round it. If so, free the cord by passing it over the baby's head. Swab the mouth and nose.
- After the head has been born, the shoulders come into anteroposterior position. Bearing down between contractions will deliver the anterior shoulder. Swing the head forward over the pubis, delivering the posterior shoulder, which will be rapidly followed by the rest of the baby.
- Turn the baby on its side to prevent aspiration. Give the mother Syntometrine (1 ml) IM after delivery. Once the cord stops pulsating, clamp it or tie it with string and cut between the ties.

*Remember*
Baby must be wrapped up warmly.

- **Normal, third-stage labour**

- With the use of Syntometrine and controlled cord traction, the placenta should be delivered within about 5 minutes. If it has not been delivered after 20 minutes, call the obstetric flying squad.
- If the placenta is retained and postpartum haemorrhage occurs, give Syntometrine (1 ml) IV and massage uterine fundus until firm. Remember that if bleeding is from a laceration it is controllable by pressure.

**Before leaving**

- consider transferring the mother and child to hospital.

### 14.1.6 The Puerperium

| *Diagnosis* | *Features* | *Management* |
|---|---|---|
| Secondary postpartum haemorrhage | Occurs 24 hours after delivery<br>Often caused by retained placental tissue | **Admit** |
| Puerperal sepsis | Infection of the genital tract<br>May be streptococcal<br>Offensive lochia | If well – take swab<br>Amoxil (500 mg) stat. and 5-day course<br>If associated bleeding **admit**<br>If unwell, feverish, toxic **admit** |
| Breast pains | Generally from engorgement<br>Rarely due to infection | Simple analgesics<br>If infected, prescribe erythromycin |
| Acute depression | May be sudden and severe<br>If mother is acutely depressed, treatment is needed not only for the mother, but also for protection of child | Urgent psychiatric opinion |

*Remember*
- Eclampsia is more likely to develop postpartum than antenatally.
- DVT and pulmonary embolism are still major causes of maternal mortality.

## 14.2 Gynaecological Emergencies

### 14.2.1 Vaginal Bleeding

- Most non-pregnant females accept bleeding as part of life and will only call if they feel that the bleeding is unusually severe or if they are worried about the possibility of serious underlying disease.

- Around puberty and the menopause, there may be flooding after a period of amenorrhoea, which may be confused with abortion.
- Menorrhagia, with heavy or prolonged bleeding, is more often dysfunctional than a symptom of organic disease.
- Intermenstrual bleeding (unless breakthrough bleeding in a woman on the contraceptive pill), post-coital and post-menopausal bleeds require careful assessment (speculum examination, VE and smear in the surgery), since they often indicate organic disease. If postmenopausal bleeding has occurred, the patient must be referred for a D & C.
- Ask for date of LMP to ensure that the patient is not pregnant.
- Ask about usual cycle, method of contraception used, apparent blood loss (number and type of pads used, any passage of clots, general condition of patient).

**See if**

- bleeding is unexpectedly severe
- general condition of the patient is not good.

**Telephone advice**

- When no need to see
  Reassure and explain the possible reason for the bleeding.
  If the bleeding is at all heavy, advise bed rest and tell the patient to make an appointment for VE, smear etc. once the bleeding has stopped.
  Ask to be called again if the bleeding becomes heavier.

- Before seeing
  *Stay lying down until seen.*

**Action when seen**

- **Assessment**

- Assess general condition, including BP and pulse.
- Perform abdominal examination and VE.

| *Assessment* | *Management* |
|---|---|
| Heavy bleeding, with any signs of shock (whatever the cause)<br>Moderate but prolonged bleeding, with risk of substantial cumulative blood loss | **Admit** |
| General condition good, but obvious pathology (e.g. fibroids, carcinoma of the cervix) | Advise bed rest<br>Arrange for appropriate further investigation and/or **referral** |
| General condition good<br>No obvious cause | Make a routine appointment once the bleeding has |

*Continued*

| *Assessment* | *Management* |
|---|---|
| | stopped for VE, speculum examination, smear, FBC and possible **referral** for investigation |

## 14.2.2 Abdominal Pain

- The general approach to assessment and management of abdominal pain is discussed on p. 100.
- This section is included purely to give a little detail about gynaecological causes of pain.

| *Diagnosis* | *Features* | *Management* |
|---|---|---|
| Acute salpingitis<br>Pyosalpinx<br>Tubo-ovarian abscess | Lower abdominal pain with tenderness; tender on VE and pelvic mass, if abscess still present. May be discharge | If not ill take endocervical swabs. Prescribe Amxyl and Flages pending results.<br>If pain severe or toxic/pyrexic **admit**<br>If abscess, **admit** |
| Dysmenorrhoea | Cramping pains in lower abdomen and back associated with menstrual flow | Soluble aspirin every 4 hours for antiprostaglandin effect<br>Apply local heat |
| Torsion of ovarian cyst, tube or pedunculated fibroid<br>Bleeding into ovarian cyst or fibroid | History of similar episodes<br>Tenderness in lower abdomen with pyrexia<br>VE reveals unilateral tender mass | **Admit** for laparotomy |
| Rupture of ovarian cyst | As torsion, but more generalised abdominal pain<br>May be shoulder pain | **Admit** for laparotomy |
| Uterovaginal prolapse | If oedematous and impossible to replace, can become very painful | **Admit** |

*Remember*
If pain is associated with any possibility of early pregnancy, consider the possibility of ectopic pregnancy.

## 14.2.3 Vaginal Discharge

- Vaginal discharge or dyspareunia is more obviously an emergency to the patient than to the doctor.

**Telephone advice**

- When no need to see
  *Attend the next surgery for examination, unless you are worried about the possibility of STD, in which case attend a special clinic.*
  If severe itch (possible thrush), advise soaking a tampon in a 50:50 mixture of white vinegar and water, and inserting tampon into vagina overnight. This will change the pH and may give some relief until can get antifungal pessaries.

## 14.2.4 Contraceptive Problems

- You may receive a panicky call for advice.

**Telephone advice**

- When no need to see
  Missed pill
  *If you are less than 12 hours late—Take missed pill now. Take next pill at normal time. Do not worry—no additional precautions needed.*

  *If you are more than 12 hours late—*
  1. *Take missed pill now. Carry on taking the rest of the pack as usual.*
     You must use a condom in addition for at least 7 days
     *AND*
  2. *Count the pills left in your packet.*
     *If there are less than 7 then start the next packet straight after you have finished this one. DO NOT HAVE THE USUAL 7 DAY BREAK.*
     *If there are 7 or more pills left, then have the usual 7 day break.*

  Breakthrough bleeding
  Reassure that the patient is still covered contraceptively.
  *Continue taking the pill. If this recurs, make a routine appointment.*

  Coil falling out
  Make sure that the patient can actually feel the coil and has not just suddenly become aware of the threads.
  If it is definitely the coil, advise her to pull gently on the thread to remove it.
  If this is painful, desist and see the patient in the surgery as soon as possible for removal.
  If the coil is successfully removed, advise the use of an alternative method of contraception until seen at a routine appointment.

  Unprotected intercourse/accident with sheath
  Reassure that morning after pill can provide protection up to 72 hours after earliest unprotected intercourse in that cycle (coil fitting will protect up to 5 days after calculated day of ovulation).
  See patient at next surgery.

# 15 Psychosocial Emergencies

*Although comparatively rare, these emergencies can be disproportionately difficult to deal with. The degree of disordered behaviour that the patient is exhibiting is more relevant to assessment and management than is a formal diagnosis.*

## Chapter Contents

## 15.1 Aberrant Behaviour

In general, society is willing to accept some unusual behaviour as normal. Different sections of society have different ideas about what constitutes normality, but once behaviour oversteps these unstated limits, the person involved will be rejected. Agencies like the police, social workers and the Samaritans may well be turned to for help, but if the behaviour is thought to be a sign of mental illness, you will be involved, whether you feel it is appropriate or not.

Although calls to acutely disturbed patients are not common, they can be very tricky to deal with and consume large amounts of time. In florid cases, a formal diagnosis may be readily made. However, making a diagnosis is not as important as assessing the behaviour of the patient and how far it is out of keeping with the circumstances. A woman smashing all the crockery in her kitchen after discovering her husband's infidelity is not mentally ill or in need of treatment. Neither is a person who is acutely distressed and weeping after a spouse's death. Yet in both cases, urgent calls may be made asking you to come and treat the person concerned. Alternatively, apparently innocuous behaviour, which is totally out of character for the individual concerned, may be a highly significant indicator of mental illness.

In many cases, it is not only the patient's mental state that you have to consider, but the mental state of the other people who have become involved, and their perceptions of abnormal behaviour. Neighbours, social workers and so on can all put great pressure on you, which must be resisted until you have properly assessed the situation for yourself. You must also firmly resist being manipulated into attempting to solve the problem, when that task may well be the responsibility of others.

Careful planning, a deal of tact, an ability to see the funny side of things, and downright low cunning are all more necessary for the resolution of these problems than are any purely medical considerations.

To summarise:

- Formal diagnosis is not as important as assessing the degree of disturbance that the patient is causing and how far it is out of keeping with the circumstances.
- In many situations, aberrant behaviour is understandable in terms of reaction to events in the patient's life, and is not a sign of mental illness.
- The mental state and reactions of other people who have become involved with the patient are always very relevant.
- Resist being manipulated or emotionally blackmailed into taking the entire responsibility for a problem, at least until you have had a chance to assess fully what is going on.
- Be careful about labelling someone as 'mad' if there is any reasonable doubt.

### 15.1.1 Differential Diagnosis and General Approach

| *Behaviour* | *Diagnosis* | *Characteristics* |
|---|---|---|
| Confusion<br>Delirium | Drugs or alcohol abuse<br>Cerebral arteriosclerosis with underlying organic complaint<br>Consider the possibility of hypoglycaemia | Disorientated in time and place<br>May be acute restlessness and panic, usually with lucid intervals<br>May be hallucinations, especially visual<br>Generally worse at night, especially in the elderly who may be found wandering |
| Aggression<br>Violence | Psychopathic behaviour<br>Drugs or alcohol abuse<br>Epilepsy or schizophrenia<br>Consider the possibility of hypoglycaemia | Usually a known personality trait and history of aggression<br>Whatever the cause, alcohol may be the precipitating factor<br>May be part of an hysterical reaction |
| Psychotic<br>Mad | Schizophrenia | Usually occurs in the young<br>Patient may have lapsed from treatment<br>Paranoid delusions<br>Auditory hallucinations<br>Totally bizarre behaviour<br>Dangerous to self and others |
| | Mania | Easy to diagnose<br>Excess activity<br>Elated mood<br>Infectious gaiety<br>May be erotically preoccupied<br>No insight<br>Not violent, unless restrained |
| | Depression | May be retarded or agitated with delusions<br>Unable to concentrate<br>Early waking<br>Depression worse in the morning<br>Guilt ridden, with consequent risk of suicide |
| Suicide threat or attempt | Temperamentally unstable | Usually young females taking tablets<br>May be an attempt to manipulate people, and the result of a family row and/or alcohol<br>Generally, others are nearby, and the patient publicises the event |
| | Mentally ill | Usually patient is middle-aged or older<br>Method attempted may shed light on the seriousness of the attempt |

*Continued*

| *Behaviour* | *Diagnosis* | *Characteristics* |
|---|---|---|
| | | May use more than one method<br>Do not publicise what they are doing, and make sure that they are alone and uninterrupted |
| Acute anxiety<br>Panic attacks<br>Hysteria<br>Situational crises | Neurosis, rarely psychosis | Usually long-standing neurotic<br>More of an emergency for the patient than the doctor<br>May be the reaction to a family row<br>Demanding, unreasonable and dependent patient and relatives<br>Patient often destroys objects<br>Overbreathing prominent<br>May present with physical symptoms |
| Bereavement<br>Grief | Normal behaviour | Acute grief with sadness, distress (physical and emotional), weeping, insomnia etc. is not a pathological process and should not be treated as such |

*Remember*
Drugs or alcohol may precipitate, or cause, most of the above kinds of behaviour.

**Telephone advice**

- Previous knowledge of the patient and the past behaviour pattern will greatly help in deciding your actions.
- With an unknown patient, the main telephone decision is whether 'madness' or an understandable emotional outburst is involved.
- Particularly in situations involving hysterical or neurotic patients, a physical symptom (headache, dizziness, weakness, apparently severe pain) may be the presenting feature. Therefore, it may be difficult to assess without seeing the patient.
- If obviously bizarre or dangerous behaviour is being exhibited or the caller is distraught, say that you are coming. This should allow further questions to be tolerated.
- On the telephone, radiate calm and sympathetic understanding, and give firm advice.

| | |
|---|---|
| • Confusion<br>Delirium | *Everyone stay calm. Do not argue with or do anything else to stimulate the patient until I arrive.* |
| • Aggression<br>Violence | Do not put yourself into danger. Consider whether police are needed with or instead of you before advising the caller. |
| • Psychotic<br>Mad | *Everyone keep calm until I arrive.* |

| | |
|---|---|
| • Suicide attempt | *If tablets have been taken take the patient direct to A & E for treatment. Take bottle or sample of tablets with you.*<br>or<br>*Stay with the patient until seen.* |
| • Suicide threat | *Stay with the patient until seen.* or if this is a known behaviour pattern, obviously temper<br>*Make an appointment for the next surgery.* |
| • Acute anxiety<br>Hysteria<br>Situational crisis | *Everyone calm down. Try ignoring the patient if he or she is acting hysterically. Medical intervention is probably not necessary.*<br>Also discuss with the caller how he or she thinks you can be of help and consider advising the patient to take an appropriate dose of psychotropic drugs that may have been previously prescribed. |
| • Bereavement<br>Grief | Calmly but firmly explain that this is a normal reaction requiring sympathy and support from relatives and friends, not drugs from the doctor. |

*Remember*

- In many situations, even if a visit is not medically necessary, the pressures from the caller may be overwhelming and a visit will have to be made to satisfy the caller, rather than you or the patient.
- In some emotional crises the family may be at breaking point and your presence, by itself, may help to resolve the situation.

**Action when seen**

**• Assessment**

- Usually fairly obvious what is, or has been, going on.
- If entry barred to you, do not break in without 'official' help, preferably from the police.
- If patient is homicidal, armed or aggressive, keep well out of reach and call the police.
- Objective is to diagnose patient's mental state and discover what has precipitated the crisis.
- If at night, ensure that there is adequate light.
- Physical examination especially important in confused elderly patients.

**• Management**

- As far as possible, act kindly, firmly and impartially.
- Do not appear to side with the relatives or those in attendance.
- Unless the patient is wildly excited, try to interview alone, listening quietly so that tension is dissipated and patient develops confidence in you.

- If possible, perform physical examination to establish your medical identity and authority; to ensure that there is no organic basis for behaviour; to allow time to consider further action.
- Do not humour patient, but allow his or her views while, without making an issue of it, expecting the patient to allow you yours.
- If you feel the need to say something, be brief, direct, honest and decisive in your statements.
- If psychiatric admission is indicated, say so; do not tell the patient lies.
- Do not chase, fight or struggle with the patient unless sufficient help is at hand to ensure relatively easy and painless victory.
- If no drugs, or only oral drugs, are needed, so much the better, but if needed parenterally ensure that sufficient help is at hand, and give IM in a large enough dose.
- Do not allow yourself to be manipulated or blackmailed into taking inappropriate action.
- Be prepared to leave if you do not feel that your help is necessary.
- If situation difficult to contain but admission not appropriate then involve local Mental Health or Crisis Intervention team.
- If admission is necessary and patient will not go voluntarily, do not try lengthy persuasion: section thus avoiding the reluctant volunteers who will promptly discharge themselves.

## 15.1.2 The Confused or Delirious Patient

- If from drugs and/or alcohol, there may be no treatment indicated other than ensuring that those in attendance keep an eye on the patient overnight.
- Demands to have an elderly patient 'taken away' are not appropriately dealt with as an emergency.
- Remember that an episode of confusion may be the only presenting symptom of many organic illnesses (e.g. heart failure, CVA, pneumonia, hypoglycaemia).

**● Management**

- As far as possible psychotropic drugs are best avoided; they may make matters worse.
- However, if patient is restless and uncontrollable, give Haloperidol (2.5–5 mg) oral or IM; in frail elderly (1.25–2.5 mg)
- Treat any underlying organic illness.
- Advise those in attendance to keep patient's bedroom well lit and to move slowly to avoid startling the patient.

**Admission** will only add to the patient's confusion, and is best avoided.

**Admit if**

- patient lives in poor social conditions
- patient lives alone
- patient requires treatment for organic illness.

Confused patients, living alone, can pose many problems, with demands for action from neighbours and relatives who cannot tolerate the abnormal behaviour, yet will not help support the patient.

The problem is heightened if
- psychogeriatric bed is unavailable
- social services are unwilling to admit the patient to Part III accommodation as an emergency
- criteria for sectioning are not fulfilled (even if sectionable, there is no guarantee a bed will be available).

*Remember*
- The police have the power to remove to a place of safety a patient found wandering.

**Before leaving**
- arrange to see a patient again for reassessment of physical and mental condition
- review social help being given by community services
- consider if patient needs domiciliary psychogeriatric assessment.
- Remember because of haloperidol's extrapyramidal side-effects thioridazine (Melleril) might be prefered if you wish to give a prescription for neuroleptic medication. Start at 10 mg BD or TID in the frail elderly (or 0.5 mg haloperidol BD—in liquid form).

### 15.1.3 The Aggressive or Violent Patient

- Requires planned approach with help of the police.
- Patient may take oral medication, but, if this is refused and the patient remains disturbed and violent, IM drug should be given while patient is restrained by others.

**● Management**
- Haloperidol (10 mg) IM
  NB: If patient is over 60, give half dose.

**Admit if**
- aggression is psychiatric in origin and patient is not taken into police custody.

**Remember**

The patient may need to be sectioned. Ensure that the hospital can cope with aggressive patients.

## 15.1.4 The Acutely Psychotic Patient

| *Assessment* | *Management* |
|---|---|
| Acute relapse schizophrenia<br>Acute mania | Give Haloperidol (10 mg) oral or IM, if needed (can repeat in 1 hour if necessary)<br>NB: If patient is over 60, give half dose<br>If admission necessary and patient does not consent, section.<br>If admission not necessary then arrange for follow-up in a few hours—refer to local mental health team. |
| Depressive psychosis | If severe, with suicide risk or agitation and delusions, arrange for emergency admission |

*Remember*
With some manic or schizophrenic patients, doses of haloperidol well in excess of those recommended may be necessary to achieve sedation. Severly disturbed patients may require an initial dose of up to 30 mg.

## 15.1.5 The Suicidal Patient

| *Assessment* | *Behaviour* | *Management* |
|---|---|---|
| Temperamentally unstable | Taken overdose | A & E for washout and/or **admission** |
| | Slashed wrists etc. | Assess significance, but do not dismiss lightly<br>May need short **admission** |
| | Issued threats | Assess significance<br>If no depressive illness, tell those in attendance to watch overnight and contact you next working day<br>Remind them that that patient not 'mad' and is responsible for own actions |
| Mentally ill | Taken overdose | **Admit** via A & E |
| | Slashed wrists etc. | **Admit** to psychiatric unit |
| | Issued threats | Take very seriously<br>May be possible to start anti-depressants and monitor at home, but, if severely depressed, urgent psychiatric opinion and/or **admission** indicated |

*Remember*
Even when the patient is obviously temperamentally unstable, exercise great caution before publicly dismissing the suicide threat, as you will then be blamed for whatever the patient does next. Do remind everyone about where responsibility lies i.e. with the patient.

### 15.1.6 The Acutely Anxious Patient

- Your calming influence may obviate the need for any therapy.

| | |
|---|---|
| • **Management** | • Diazepam (10 mg) oral or IM, if needed |

### 15.1.7 The Patient in a Situational Crisis

- Your calming influence should obviate the need for any therapy.
- Reassure everyone that there is no danger of mental illness.
- Ask what help is required of you and do not be manipulated into sorting out the problem, other than at a later time and place more convenient to you.
- If patient will not allow situation to settle, and continues to act out, it may be necessary to warn that if patient insists on acting mad then may be treated as such.

| | |
|---|---|
| • **Management** | • Diazepam (10 mg) oral or IM, if needed |

### 15.1.8 The Grieving Patient

- Listen, and reassure everyone that the feelings being experienced are normal.
- Resist prescribing, but, if pressured, prescribe a mild hypnotic, only for a few nights.

## 15.2 Admission of a Patient Under Compulsion

### 15.2.1 England and Wales

- Only patients who cannot be persuaded to enter hospital voluntarily can be admitted under compulsion.
- Compulsion should never be used lightly, and good notes must be kept in case of later legal complications.
- Compulsion can be used when a patient suffers from a mental disorder that warrants detention in hospital, either when treatment is necessary in the interests of the patient's own health or when detention is necessary for the patient's safety or the safety of others. NB: It is not essential that there be danger to self or others.
- If the patient is sectioned without the consent of the relatives, no come back is possible if certification was carried out 'in good faith'.

- If enforced sedation was given 'in good faith' prior to admission, legal repercussions are unlikely, although a social worker may be unwilling to sign an application if the patient was sedated before his or her arrival.
- Section 2 (assessment) should be used where possible, but in most general practice emergencies section 4 (emergency) is far more appropriate.

Section 4 (emergency)—Maximum length of compulsory admission: 72 hours.

(a) Applied for by an approved social worker for the nearest relative.
(b) Supported by medical recommendation made by one doctor who, if practicable, should have previous knowledge of the patient.
(c) Applicant and doctor must have seen the patient in the last 24 hours.
(d) Patient must be admitted within 24 hours, or earlier, of application or medical recommendation.
(e) Acceptance by a receiving hospital is necessary—sectioning does not guarantee your patient's admission.

Section 2 (assessment)—Maximum length of compulsory admission: 28 days.

(a) Applied for by an approved social worker or nearest relative.
(b) Supported by medical recommendations from 2 doctors including one approved under S12 and, if practicable, one with knowledge of the patient.
(c) Maximum time allowed between examination by the 2 doctors is 5 days.
(d) Patient has right to a Mental Health Review Tribunal in the first 14 days.
(e) Acceptance by the receiving hospital is necessary.

*Remember*
For admission under section 2 or 4

- in many cases, the patient can be left with relatives who can also keep the Mental Health Act form (from your bag and which you have filled in) until the social worker arrives. This leaves you free to go home to telephone to arrange for admission
- relationships in order of precedence are: husband or wife; son or daughter; father; mother; brother or sister; grandparent; grandchild; uncle or aunt; nephew or niece.

The relative with whom the patient 'ordinarily resides' or from whom care is received is held to be the nearest. A person with whom an unmarried, deserted or separated patient has been living for at least 5 years is deemed to be a relative.

## 15.2.2 Scotland

- In an emergency, use section 31 of the Mental Health (Scotland) Act 1960:

(a) One signature must be obtained from a doctor who has examined the patient that day.
(b) You must try to obtain the consent of a relative or mental officer to the admission. If this is not possible, you must state why.
(c) Patient can be detained for 7 days.

## 15.2.3 Northern Ireland

- In an emergency, use Admission Form 3 of the Mental Health (Northern Ireland) Act 1961 (sections 12, 13, 14 and 15 cover compulsory admission).

(a) Part 1 of the form is the application, which may be signed by any relative or a social worker.
(b) Part 2 of the form is the medical recommendation, which must state the date on which the patient was examined and contain a clinical description of the patient's mental condition, on which the doctor's opinion of why the patient is mentally ill to such a degree that he or she needs to be detained in hospital, is based. It must also state why informal admission is not suitable.
(c) Part 3 of the form is a statement of the particulars of the patient.
(d) The relevant psychiatric hospital must be contracted.
(e) The patient may be detained for 7 days.

This emergency procedure is only to be used where there would be an undesirable delay if one were to comply with section 13 of the Act.

## Notes

# 16 Respiratory Emergencies

*The predominant emergency symptom presented by the major respiratory illnesses is acute or severe breathlessness.*

*Although essentially cardiovascular conditions, acute LVF and pulmonary embolism also present as acute breathlessness. Accordingly, their main features are included in the differential diagnosis of breathlessness, while their management is discussed in the chapter on the cardiovascular system.*

*Pneumothorax, pneumonia, pleurisy and tracheitis may also present as chest pain. Their management is discussed in this chapter, though they are also included in the differential diagnosis of chest pain (p. 52).*

## Chapter Contents

# 16.1 Acute Breathlessness

Acute breathlessness is a frightening symptom for both the patient and those in attendance. Although the large majority of patients who complain of breathlessness are suffering from an organic disease, the degree of the subjective feeling of breathlessness bears no constant relationship to the degree of functional abnormality.

Assessing the degree of urgency over the telephone is difficult and often an immediate visit will be necessary. However, if it is possible that a foreign body has been inhaled, telephone advice may be lifesaving.

Remember that breathlessness without clear physical signs is likely to be organic in origin, unless there are obvious features of hyperventilation. The ketotic diabetic may present with breathlessness.

## 16.1.1 Differential Diagnosis

| *Complaint* | *Characteristics* | *Physical signs* |
|---|---|---|
| Asthma | Sudden onset<br>May be triggered by URTI, exertion, allergens or emotion<br>Usually a history of previous attacks<br>May be atopic history | Hyperinflated chest<br>Decreased movement of chest, decreased PEFR<br>Wheezing, mainly expiratory<br>NB: In a severe attack the chest may be silent<br>Tachycardia |
| Acute exacerbation of chronic bronchitis or emphysema | Long 'bronchitic' history<br>Cough producing purulent sputum<br>Fever<br>Malaise | Hyperinflated chest<br>Decreased movement of chest<br>Wheezing |
| Pneumonia | Can occur in chronically ill, or fit and healthy<br>URTI, followed by cough, fever, pleuritic pain | Affected side exhibits: decreased movement; dullness on percussion; decreased breath sounds; creps.; ± rub |
| Hyperventilation | Anxiety, with disproportionate breathlessness<br>Distraction, lightheadedness, with paraesthesiae of extremities | Upper sternal heaving but relative lack of costal expansion |
| Acute laryngeal obstruction | Result of oedema or inhalation of foreign body<br>Severe distress<br>Stridor | Enormous, but ineffective, respiratory efforts |

*Continued*

| *Complaint* | *Characteristics* | *Physical signs* |
|---|---|---|
| Spontaneous pneumothorax | Occurs mainly in young, lanky males<br>Sudden breathlessness<br>May be unilateral chest pain, though often painless | Affected side exhibits:<br>decreased movement;<br>hyperresonance;<br>decreased breath sounds;<br>possible tracheal shift away<br>NB: Signs are not reliable and may not be present |
| Acute LVF | Occurs mainly in older patients<br>Abrupt onset often at night<br>Possible complication of myocardial infarction<br>Orthopnoea<br>Possibly blood-flecked, frothy sputum | Masses of fine creps.<br>NB: In the early stages there may be no signs in the chest<br>Tachycardia |
| Pulmonary embolism | If massive, then shock and collapse<br>Otherwise, haemoptysis and pleuritic pain<br>Often history of unexplained, mild attacks of dyspnoea; ask for this if diagnosis is being considered | If pulmonary infarction, signs as for pneumonia<br>May be evidence of DVT<br>Tachycardia |

Patient can be rapidly assessed on the basis of

- character and rate of respiration
- any signs of shock
- presence or absence of cyanosis, use of accessory muscles, hyperinflated chest.

## 16.1.2 Asthma

- Potentially fatal disease, the severity of which is consistently underestimated by both GPs and patients.
- Characteristic exacerbations and remissions of reversible airways obstruction.
- Reversibility is not necessarily immediate, even with intensive therapy.
- Predominant symptom is breathlessness, associated with expiratory wheezing.
- Pain is not a feature.
- Usually a history of similar attacks, often dating from childhood.
- Before contacting you, most patients will have used bronchodilator drugs without gaining relief.
- When airways are acutely obstructed beyond a certain point, inhaled treatment will not work; systemic therapy is then necessary.

- Patients who use a steroid inhaler and have developed a severe attack, or a moderate attack which fails to respond readily to bronchodilator therapy, must take oral prednisolone immediately.

**See unless**

- patient can talk to you without effort **and**
- patient has not properly used available drugs.

**Telephone advice**

- When no need to see
  *Sit down and try to relax. Use 3 puffs of the inhaler (UNLESS intal or steroid). If there is no improvement in 1 hour, call again and I will see you.*

- Before seeing
  *Sit up and lean forward. Try to relax, and I will see you as soon as possible.*
- If uncertain of the diagnosis, consider acute LVF, especially if the patient is middle-aged or elderly.

**Action when seen**

- **Assessment**

| *Asthma* | *Acute LVF* |
|---|---|
| Often long history of episodic attacks of breathlessness | Usually first attack of breathlessness often in middle-age or later |
| Marked wheezing | Wheezing less marked |
| Sputum may be thick or purulent | Sputum may be frothy and blood-stained |
| Expiratory rhonchi | Basal creps. |
| Possible pulsus paradoxus | Possible pulsus alternans, triple rhythm |
| Generally healthy CVS | May be signs of underlying heart disease |

- Assess severity of attack

| *Mild attack* | *Severe attack* |
|---|---|
| Patient can speak and move | Patient too breathless to speak or move |
| Audible expiratory wheezing | Chest may be silent because insufficient air movement to cause wheezing |
| Diffuse rhonchi on auscultation | |
| Poor chest expansion | Gross thoracic overinflation, with use of all accessory muscles of respiration |
| Healthy colour | Pale, severely distressed, cyanosed |
| Pulse: less than 110 and regular | Pulse: more than 130 and paradoxical |
| Peak flow rate: 200 or more | Peak flow rate: 100 or less |

**Danger signs**

- inability to talk or stand
- cyanosis
- chest quiet on auscultation
- pulse over 130 and/or paradoxical
- increasing restlessness and confusion.

**● Management**

- Confident attitude and firm, decisive action are vital to reassure the patient.

*Remember*

- NEVER give sedatives during an attack, even if anoxia makes the patient confused or aggressive.
- The Volumatic has been shown to be as effective as a nebuliser, however a nebuliser is sometimes useful in very young or elderly patients who cannot or will not use a spacer properly.

---

Mild attack

Use 4–8 puffs Salbutamol inhaler by Volumatic
Check patient is using inhaler correctly. Advise to use 2 puffs bronchodilator inhaler 4 hourly for next 24–48 hours, whether feels wheezy or not.
Ask to be recalled if patient worsens.

Moderate attack

Use 8 puffs Salbutamol inhaler by Volumatic (repeat in 10 minutes if necessary). Alternatively 2.5 mg (2.5 ml) Salbutamol by nebuliser.
Start prednisolone 40 mg oral daily for 5 days
Do not leave the patient until you are certain the attack has remitted—if not much improved in 20–30 minutes **admit.**
Reassess after 4 hours, but make sure you are called before this if the wheezing starts again.

Severe Attack, or if **danger signs** present

Use 16 puffs Salbutamol inhaler by Volumatic or 0.5 mg by nebuliser
Start dose of Prednisolone 60 mg or Hydrocortisone (300 mg) IV
**Admit** to hospital by ambulance, with oxygen.

---

**Admit if**

- severe attack or **danger signs** present
- prolonged attack, without remission
- attack complicated by pneumothorax
- moderate attack which does not respond to therapy
- patient or family obviously wish it
- you are not confident of coping with patient.

If there is any doubt whatsoever regarding the safety of the patient, err on the side of caution and **admit.** Too many young people still die because of failure of early admission.

**Before leaving**

- ensure that you will be called if the patient worsens or inhaler has had no effect

- tell patient to make an early appointment to allow reassessment of general lines of long-term management.
- remember there is a case for advising asthmatics to go directly to A & E when they feel that an attack is about to become severe.

## 16.1.3 Chest Infection

Bronchitis and pneumonia will present with a story of fever, cough, breathlessness and possibly chest pain. In the elderly, confusion may be the main feature.

### 16.1.3.1 Acute Exacerbation of Chronic Obstructive Pulmonary Disease

- Patient has long 'bronchitic' history.
- Generally, patient is already on bronchodilator and, possibly, antibiotic therapy.
- Patient has cough with purulent sputum, increasing breathlessness (which, like LVF, may be worsened by lying down), fever, malaise.
- Often initiated by URTI.
- May be accompanied by right-sided heart failure (cor pulmonale).

**Visit unless**

- patient has been seen recently, is on appropriate therapy, and his or her condition is well known to you.

**Telephone advice**

- Before seeing
  *Keep patient comfortable until I arrive.*

**Action when seen**

- **Assessment**
  - The degree of respiratory distress is a good indication of the severity of the attack.
  - Coarse creps. and rhonchi, mainly at the bases, are characteristic.
  - General bronchospasm may mimic late asthma.
  - Elevated JVP, hepatomegaly and sacral and/or ankle oedema signify right-sided heart failure.

- **Management**

For infection
  Oral, broad-spectrum antibiotic.

For bronchospasm
  4–8 puffs of Ventolin inhaler by Volumatic
  If severe, see Asthma (p. 161)

For respiratory failure
  Oxygen at 24%, if available.
  If patient confused and restless, **Admit.**

For right-sided heart failure
  Frusemide (40 mg) oral.
  If severe, **Admit.**

**Admit if**

- patient shows signs of significant respiratory failure developing
- patient has severe or worsening heart failure
- patient lives alone or in poor social conditions.

**Before leaving**

- decide whether to revisit after a suitable interval, or whether patient may be seen at routine appointment.

### 16.1.3.2 Pneumonia

- Clinical condition is more important than type (lobar or bronchopneumonia).
- May be preterminal event in chronically ill patients.
- May affect the young and fit, in which case more likely to be viral than bacterial.
- Infecting agent unlikely to be identified.
- Generally characterised by URTI, followed by productive cough, breathlessness and pleuritic pain.
- Confusion may be only symptom in elderly.

**See unless**

- patient is terminally ill, known to you, and taking appropriate analgesics.

**Telephone advice**

- Before seeing
  *Keep patient comfortable until seen.*

**Action when seen**

- **Assessment**

- Patient breathless, pyrexial, hypoxic, possibly confused.
- Elderly patient may be apyrexial.
- Patient may exhibit clinical signs of consolidation or area of coarse creps. or rhonchi.

- **Management**

- Amoxil (500 mg) oral or IM stat., and prescription for (250 mg) TDS for 7 days.
- Paracetamol or soluble aspirin every 4 hours.
- Hot lemon drinks.

**Admit if**

- patient is in significant respiratory distress
- patient lives alone or in poor social conditions.

In preterminal patients, circumstances could arise in which any treatment might be considered inappropriate.

**Before leaving**

- arrange to reassess patient in 24–48 hours
- consider whether chest X-ray is necessary for diagnostic purposes, to check progress or to exclude underlying carcinoma.

*Remember*
If the patient shows no improvement in 48 hours, you may need to change the antibiotic to erythromycin or tetracycline. If clinically worse—admit.

## 16.1.4 Hyperventilation

- Usually easily recognised, if considered as diagnosis rather than symptom.
- Affects both sexes.
- Pain triggers vicious circle of anxiety and hyperventilation.
- Paradoxically, most striking symptom is dyspnoea.
- Patient is very anxious, distracted and light-headed.
- Patient may have paraesthesiae of extremities and round the mouth.
- Patient may have carpopedal spasm or generalised tetany.

**See unless**

- this is a known behaviour pattern of the patient and you can allay the caller's anxiety so that they can cope effectively.

**Telephone advice**

- When no need to see
  *Everyone keep calm. Get the patient to hold breath and then breathe as slowly as possible, or to rebreathe into a paper bag.*
- Before seeing
  *Everyone keep calm. Get the patient to breathe slowly.*

**Action when seen**

- **Assessment**
  - Patient's anxiety is usually shared by those in attendance.
  - Pallor and tachycardia.
  - Possible carpopedal spasm, generalised tetany, or faintness.
  - Disproportionate breathlessness.
  - Upper sternal heaving but relative lack of coastal expansion.
  - Examination should quickly rule out asthma, LVF, respiratory obstruction.
- **Management**
  - Be calm and reassuring.
  - Tell patient to take shallower and slower breaths.
  - Tell patient to rebreathe into paper bag.
  - Response to management will confirm diagnosis.

**Before leaving**

- ensure that everyone understands what has been happening.

## 16.1.5 Acute laryngeal obstruction

### 16.1.5.1 Inhalation of a Foreign Body

- Usually occurs while patient is eating or, in children, during play.
- Most foreign bodies pass through the vocal cords and lodge in the lower airway, in which cases symptoms will be less acute.
- Patient often instinctively clutches throat with hands.
- If airway completely obstructed, patient is unable to speak or breathe, becomes pale, then rapidly cyanosed and finally loses consciousness and collapses.

*Remember*
Death or brain damage will occur within 4 minutes if urgent action is not taken.

**Telephone advice**

- **The caller must appreciate that successful action is his responsibility. Calm the caller and quickly give clear, easily followed instructions.**

*Stand behind the patient and encircle the waist with your arms. With one hand, make a fist and place it, thumb-side first, against the patient's stomach, slightly above the navel. Grasp the fist with your other hand and press into the patient's stomach with a quick upward thrust. This has to be forceful to blow the food blocking the windpipe right out. It may be necessary to repeat the thrust up to six times to clear the airway.*

*For child or baby:*
As above, sitting the child on lap and using less force for thrust. For baby, use middle and index fingers of both hands instead of fist.

WAIT TO HEAR OUTCOME.

If thrusts fail to clear airway:
*Try to hook out object or push it right down using finger.*

**See**

- whether telephone advice is successful or not
- if inhaled foreign body is suspected, even if no symptoms present.

**Action when seen**

- **Management**

| | |
|---|---|
| If any suspicion that foreign body was inhaled | **Refer** at once to A & E or ENT |
| If actual respiratory obstruction | As telephone advice |
| If this action has failed | Push large-bore needle (medicut) through cricothyroid membrane<br>**Admit,** accompanying patient to hospital in ambulance |

*Remember*
A choking patient will die without your intervention, and so has nothing to lose by your efforts.

### 16.1.5.2 Angioneurotic Oedema

- Result of local or anaphylactic shock.
- May be reaction to drugs, insect stings or ingested food.
- Patient suffers itching, bronchospasm, cyanosis and collapse.
- Unless treatment available within minutes, patient is likely to die.

**Telephone advice**
- Depending on distances involved
  Dial 999 for ambulance or, if quicker, take patient to A & E by car.

**Action when seen**
(if you reach patient before ambulance)
- **Assessment**
  - Oedema of face, glottis and larynx.
  - Rapid, thready pulse.
- **Management**
  - Lie patient flat and elevate the feet.
  - Adrenaline (epinephrine) (0.5 ml) 1 in 1000 IM (repeat after 5 minutes if no response).
  - Piriton (10–20 mg) IM or IV.
  - Hydrocortisone (200 mg) IV.
  - **Admit** in ambulance, with oxygen.

## 16.1.6 Spontaneous Pneumothorax

- Occurs mainly in young, healthy, lanky males.
- May be recurrent.
- Generally presents with acute, unilateral, pleuritic-like chest pain and breathlessness, or breathlessness alone.
- If small, may be symptomless, unless there is pre-existing obstructive airways disease; chest X-ray may be the only means of diagnosis.
- May complicate asthma or LVF.
- Rarely, the pleural tear may act as a one-way valve, resulting in a potentially lethal increase in intrapleural pressure (tension pneumothorax).

**See**

**Telephone advice**
- Before seeing
  *Sit up, leaning forward, until seen.*

**Action when seen**
- **Assessment**

| *Small pneumothorax* | *Large pneumothorax* | *Tension pneumothorax* |
|---|---|---|
| Some dyspnoea | Dyspnoea and distress | Extreme respiratory distress |
| May be some pain | May be some pain or tearing feeling | |
| Healthy colour | Possible cyanosis | Cyanosis |
| Examination may prove negative | Affected side exhibits: diminished movement of chest; hyperresonance; diminished breath sounds | Gross mediastinal displacement<br>Trachea shifted away from pneumothorax |
| Pulse: normal | Tachycardia | Pulse: rapid, small volume |
| BP: normal | BP: steady | BP: falling |

*Remember*
Pain is not a constant feature and, in itself, is not a reliable indication of the size of the pneumothorax.

- **Management**
  - Small or large pneumothorax
    Temgesic (0.2–0.4 mg) SL for pain.
    **Admit,** because of significant risk of potentially lethal tension pneumothorax developing.
  - Tension pneumothorax
    Insert wide-bore needle (medicut) *via* the 2nd and 3rd interspace in mid-clavicular line on affected side.
    Temgesic (0.4 mg) SL
    **Admit,** accompanying patient to hospital in ambulance with oxygen.

## 16.2 Cough

- Emergency call most often from parents of children with URTI.
- If acute, ensure that it is not due to inhalation of a foreign body.

**See if**

- there is the possibility that a foreign body has been inhaled
- patient has associated breathlessness or chest pain
- patient appears to be ill.

**Telephone advice**

- When no need to see
  *Take hot lemon drink.*

## 16.3 Haemoptysis

- Frightening symptom, only rarely having a serious cause.
- May be doubt as to whether haematemesis or haemoptysis.
- Generally result of rupture of superficial tracheal veins by strenuous coughing.
- May result from infection, neoplasm or pulmonary embolism.

**See if**

- bleeding appears to be brisk
- patient appears to be ill or in shock
- patient has associated dyspnoea or chest pain
- telephone reassurance is not readily accepted.

**Telephone advice**

- When no need to see
  *Hot lemon drink will ease cough. Make appointment for next working day. Call me back if other symptoms develop.*
- Before seeing
  *Sit upright and loosen collar. Collect any phlegm before seen.*

**Action when seen**

- **Assessment**
  - Confirm haemoptysis and not haematemesis.
  - Assess general state of patient.
  - Perform full ENT and chest examination, check for finger clubbing.
  - Check legs for possible DVT.

- **Management**

| *Assessment* | *Management* |
|---|---|
| Moderate bleeding from any cause | **Admit** |
| Acute chest infection | See p. 162 |
| Pulmonary embolism | See p. 53 |
| Suspected neoplasm or TB | Investigate routinely |

**Before leaving**

- if diagnosis is not obvious, advise patient that further investigation will be necessary
- ask patient to make routine appointment.

## 16.4 Hiccups

- Usually an isolated, benign, self-limiting condition.
- May be symptom of chronic or serious disease (e.g. chronic renal failure, peritonitis), in which case likely to be intractable.
- Call for advice is likely only if they are persistent and painful.

**See if**

- hiccups are severe, distressing or very persistent
- hiccups appear to be the result of underlying disease requiring assessment.

**Telephone advice**

- When no need to see
  *Try folk remedies (hold breath; eat large spoonful of sugar)*

**Action when seen**

- Assess and treat any underlying condition.
- For persistent distressing hiccups, Haloperidol (2.5–5 mg) IM or oral may help.

## 16.5 Influenza

- Strictly speaking, refers to epidemic influenza caused by the influenza subgroup of the myxoviruses, but the diagnosis is used by both doctors and patients for feverish URTIs seldom due to any specific virus.
- In epidemics, prevalence is highest in children and young adults.
- Complications are more likely in the elderly.
- Patient suffers sudden onset of malaise, fever, cough, coryza, aching and sweating, lasting 2–3 days and followed by gradual improvement.
- Most cases are uncomplicated and benign, but there is a case fatality rate of 1 per 500 patients.

*Remember*
Malaria cases are often wrongly diagnosed as influenza.

**See if**

- patient is elderly and already suffering from chronic cardiac or respiratory condition
- patient has not improved after 3 or 4 days
- patient has increasingly productive cough or breathlessness.

**Telephone advice**

- When no need to see
  *Stay in bed. Take hot lemon drinks. Take aspirin or paracetamol every 4 hours. I will visit if the symptoms persist for 3 or 4 days without improvement.*

- Before seeing
  *Keep comfortable until seen.*

**Action when seen**

- As for acute chest infection p. 162

**Notes**

# 17 Urogenital Emergencies

*Symptoms of urinary tract infection are the commonest reason for an emergency call in this system. However, haematuria, testicular pain and failure to pass urine are all dramatic occurrences which will result in early seeking of medical help.*

## Chapter Contents

## 17.1 Balanitis

- Infection of the space between the foreskin and the penis.
- Characterised by soreness, redness of the foreskin or glans, and a discharge, which is usually profuse.
- Do not confuse with paraphimosis or with red ammoniacal foreskin resulting from nappy rash.
- Majority of cases occur in young boys.
- If in the older male, exclude STD, diabetes and carcinoma of the penis.

**Telephone advice**

- When no need to see
  *Give the patient a suitable analgesic. Apply a bland antiseptic cream. Make a routine appointment.*

## 17.2 Haematuria

- Important symptom of urinary tract infection.
- Alarms patients and causes them to seek urgent advice.
- Normal urine colour can vary greatly; redness may be caused by beetroot or laxative.
- Associated frequency, urgency and dysuria suggest infection, which is the most common cause.
- Renal colic preceding bleeding suggests the presence of a stone, but following bleeding suggests neoplasm.
- If painless, more likely to have a serious underlying cause.
- Further investigation is essential.

**See if**

- blood clots are being passed
- patient appears to be ill or shocked
- patient is in moderate pain
- haematuria is within 2 weeks of injury
- telephone reassurance is not readily accepted.

**Telephone advice**

- When no need to see
  *Drink extra fluids. Tests must be carried out, so make appointment for next working day. Bring a urine sample to the appointment.*

- Before seeing
  *Collect any urine passed before seen.*

**Action when seen**

- **Assessment**
  - Confirm diagnosis and ascertain precise nature of bleeding.
  - Take BP and pulse to gauge severity of bleeding.
  - Check that the bladder is not distended.

● **Management**

| *Assessment* | *Management* |
|---|---|
| Moderate bleeding from any cause | **Admit** |
| Possibility of traumatic origin | **Admit** |
| Renal colic | See p. 175 |
| Urinary tract infection | See p. 177 |

## 17.3 Paraphimosis

- Tight ring of foreskin stuck behind the glans.
- If seen early, you may be able to help.

**Direct to A & E**

- if a young child or if contact delayed, as circumcision may be necessary

**Otherwise visit**

**Telephone advice**

- Before seeing
  *Give aspirin or paracetamol. Have a bowl filled with chips of ice ready for me. I shall be with you as soon as possible.*

**Action when seen**

● **Management**

- Loosely fill plastic bag with ice chips.
- Invaginate the penis into it for 15 minutes.
- Apply gentle forward traction on the foreskin, combined with pressure on glans.
- If unsuccessful, **refer to A & E**.

## 17.4 Retention of Urine

- Generally occurs in elderly men with prostatic hypertrophy.
- May be result of urological or non-urological mechanical obstruction (e.g. fibroids, stricture, calculi, retroverted gravid uterus).
- May be the result of drugs, hysteria or neurological condition.
- May result simply from constipation in the bedbound.
- Can occur with or without overflow incontinence.

**Telephone advice**

- Before seeing
  *If feasible, get the patient to relax in a hot bath. After 10–15 minutes, whilst still relaxing in the bath, attempt to pass urine; if this is not successful, phone back and I shall visit.*

**Action when seen**

- **Assessment**
  - Examine abdomen: distended, tender, tense bladder whose palpation initiates the desire to micturate, implies acute obstruction.
  - Perform PR.
  - Assess the general condition of the patient.

- **Management**
  - Unless retention has been caused by constipation in an elderly bedbound patient, **admission** is likely to be necessary.
  - Chronic retention with no pain is a contraindication to extrahospital catheterisation as sudden bladder decompression may lead to bleeding, hyponatraemia, hypovolaemia and shock.
  - Acute retention is painful and distressing and therefore warrants alleviation before the ambulance ride to hospital. Give Temgesic (0.2–0.4 mg) SL.

    Catheterise:

    Lubricate a small (14–16 French gauge) soft Foley catheter with KY jelly or boiled water.

    Pass under as aseptic conditions as possible.

    If there is any difficulty introducing the catheter, or if any bleeding occurs, abandon the procedure.

    Do NOT empty the whole bladder quickly.

    Pull foreskin forward after catheterisation.
  - If acute retention is caused by constipation and social conditions, home care may be possible, in which case:

    Catheterise.

    Perform manual evacuation of faeces (GP or district nurse).

    Administer suppositories or enemas (district nurse).

    Remove catheter when the constipation has cleared.

**Before leaving**

- Advise the patient who is staying at home that a nurse will call
- explain to the patient who is going to hospital what is going to happen.

## 17.5 Renal Colic

- Easily self-diagnosed by a patient who has had it before.
- Generally presents as a sudden, intense pain that starts without warning.
- Usually begins in the loin and radiates to the iliac fossa, groin and even genitalia.
- May be associated vomiting.
- If obstruction is at the lower end of the ureter or bladder, then dysuria, frequency, strangury and urgency may be experienced.
- Generally the result of calculi, but if haematuria precedes colic, suspect neoplasm.

**See**

**Telephone advice**

- Before seeing
  *Collect any urine passed before seen.*

**Action when seen**

- **Assessment**
  - Patient maybe completely incapacitated and very anxious.
  - Patient may lie very still or attempt to obtain relief by frequent changes of position.
  - Patient may appear shocked and sweating.
  - In spite of the severe symptoms, abdominal examination will characteristically reveal only some renal tenderness.
  - Urinalysis should reveal protein and blood to confirm diagnosis.

- **Management**
  - Diclofenac (75 mg) IM
  - If vomiting, Stemetil (12.5 mg) IM.
  - If no pain relief in 30 minutes, atropine (0.6 mg) SC and/or repeat Diclofenac (75 mg) IM.
  - If treating at home:
    Dihydrocodeine (30 mg) oral every 4–6 hours.
    If vomiting, Stemetil (25 mg) PR every 4–6 hours.

**Admit if**

- you are in any doubt about diagnosis and wish IVP urgently
- pain is not adequately controlled
- patient is known to have renal impairment or only one kidney
- patient lives alone or in poor conditions
- patient is febrile
- symptoms persist for more than 24 hours.

**Before leaving**

- explain the condition to help allay anxiety
- ensure that the patient increases fluid intake
- ensure that instructions regarding medication are fully understood
- advise that you will revisit after a suitable interval, but must be called earlier if the symptoms are not allayed by therapy or if the patient's urine output over the next few hours is poor.

## 17.6 Testicular Pain

### 17.6.1 Epididymo-orchitis

- Often affects the epididymis more than the testes.
- Usually associated with symptoms of lower urinary tract infection.
- Most likely caused by NSU or gonococcal infection.

### 17.6.2 Mumps Orchitis

- Affects 25% of post-pubertal mumps cases.
- Occurs within 7–10 days of onset of disease.
- Usually unilateral.
- Characterised by acute pain, tenderness and swelling of the testicle.

### 17.6.3 Torsion of the Testicle

- Generally characterised by sudden-onset of pain in the scrotum and/or groin.
- May have a more gradual onset in children.
- Often associated with vomiting.
- Commonest in children and teenagers.
- Possible history of mild episodes in the past.

**See quickly if**

- there is any suspicion of torsion (delay will put testicular viability in danger).

**Telephone advice**

- Before seen
  *Elevate and support the scrotum until seen.*

**Action when seen**

- **Assessment**

| *Torsion* | *Epididymo-orchitis* |
|---|---|
| Patient generally under 20 | Patient generally over 20 |
| Unilateral | May be bilateral |
| No urinary symptoms | May be urinary symptoms |
| Testis and epididymis tender, swollen and retracted | May be confined to epididymis |
| Testis may hang horizontally, like a bell clapper | Elevation and support of the scrotum may help relieve pain |

In the absence of a clear history of recent mumps, mumps orchitis and torsion are indistinguishable.

- **Management**

| *Assessment* | *Management* |
|---|---|
| ANY suspicion whatsoever of torsion | **Admit** |
| Mumps orchitis | Prednisolone (15 mg) oral QID for 4 days<br>Rest and scrotal support |
| Epididymo-orchitis | Rest, scrotal support and suitable analgesia<br>Treatment for NSU and/or gonorrhoea, if indicated |

**Before leaving**

- if mumps orchitis has been diagnosed, reassure the patient that there is no risk of impotence and that only the affected testicle might have its fertility impaired; the other will remain normal
- if epididymo-orchitis has been diagnosed, consider advising attendance at the next STD clinic.

## 17.7 Urinary Tract Infection

- Frequency and dysuria, possibly with haematuria, nocturia, loin and suprapubic pain, urgency and strangury, mean that the diagnosis is rarely in doubt.
- There is a variable degree of systemic upset (pyrexia, rigors, vomiting).
- May be silent, especially in the young, old or pregnant.
- Diagnosis must be considered in patients who are generally unwell and have a pyrexia or are vomiting for no obvious reason.
- More likely to affect women than men.

**See if**

- systemic upset predominates
- you suspect pyelonephritis rather than cystitis
- patient is in much discomfort or pain
- patient is pregnant, a diabetic, has calculi or has a pre-existing renal disease.

**Telephone advice**

- When no need to see
  *Drink extra fluids. Make an appointment for the next working day. Bring a urine sample to the appointment.*

- Before seeing
  *Collect any urine passed before seen.*

**Action when seen**

- **Assessment**
  - Confirm diagnosis
  - Delineate aggravating or predisposing factors.
  - Assess patient's general condition (temperature and pulse).
  - Take urinalysis specimen for sugar, protein and blood.
  - Take MSU for culture, if sterile bottle available.

- **Management**

| *Assessment* | *Management* |
|---|---|
| Lower urinary tract infection (cystitis) | Give extra fluids<br>Prescribe antibiotics |
| Upper urinary tract infection (pyelonephritis) | Amoxil (500 mg) oral or IM stat.<br>If vomiting, Stemetil (12.5 mg) IM<br>Prescribe Amoxil course |
| Moderate or severe systemic upset in the pregnant, diabetic or the patient with pre-existing renal disease or damage | **Admit** |

**Before leaving**

- remember that a revisit may be necessary if systemic upset does not improve or worsens
- if an upper urinary tract infection advise the patient that must make a routine appointment 3 days after the antibiotic course has finished, for a check MSU.

## 17.8 Sexually Transmitted Diseases

- The sudden realisation that they have an STD or that they are at risk of having caught it may cause patients to panic and call the doctor.

**Telephone advice**

- When visit not necessary
  *Attend the next STD clinic or make routine appointment.*

# Index